Baldwinsville Public Library
30 East Genesee Street
Baldwinsville, NY 13027-2575
JUL 18 2016

WITHDRAWN

ACCELERATED RECOVERY OF YOUR HEALTH

D1519213

How to recover your body after injury or surgery

HOWARD B. COTLER MD FACS FAAOS FABOS

Accelerated Recovery of Your Health: How to recover your body after injury or surgery

Copyright © 2016 Howard B. Cotler MD, FACS, FAAOS, FABOS

JUL 2 8 2016

Published by Atlantic Publishing Group, Inc.
1405 SW 6th Avenue • Ocala, Florida 34471 • Phone 800-814-1132 • Fax 352-622-1875
Website: www.atlantic-pub.com • Email: sales@atlantic-pub.com
SAN Number: 268-1250

No part of this publication may be reproduced, stored in a retrieval system, or transmitted in any form or by any means, electronic, mechanical, photocopying, recording, scanning, or otherwise, except as permitted under Section 107 or 108 of the 1976 United States Copyright Act, without the prior written permission of the Publisher. Requests to the Publisher for permission should be sent to Atlantic Publishing Group, Inc., 1405 SW 6th Ave., Ocala, Florida 34471.

Library of Congress Cataloging-in-Publication Data

Names: Cotler, H. B. (Howard B.), author.
Title: Accelerated recovery of your health : how to recover your body after
  injury or surgery / by Howard Cotler MD FACS FAAOS FABOS.
Description: Ocala, Florida : Atlantic Publishing Group, Inc., 2016. |
  Includes bibliographical references and index.
Identifiers: LCCN 2016002471| ISBN 9781620231340 (alk. paper) | ISBN 1620231344 (alk. paper)
Subjects: LCSH: Surgery--Physiological aspects. | Surgery--Popular works. |
  Self-care, Health--Popular works.
Classification: LCC RD31.7 .C68 2016 | DDC 617.001/9—dc23 LC record available at
http://lccn.loc.gov/2016002471

LIMIT OF LIABILITY/DISCLAIMER OF WARRANTY: The publisher and the author make no representations or warranties with respect to the accuracy or completeness of the contents of this work and specifically disclaim all warranties, including without limitation warranties of fitness for a particular purpose. No warranty may be created or extended by sales or promotional materials. The advice and strategies contained herein may not be suitable for every situation. This work is sold with the understanding that the publisher is not engaged in rendering legal, accounting, or other professional services. If professional assistance is required, the services of a competent professional should be sought. Neither the publisher nor the author shall be liable for damages arising herefrom. The fact that an organization or Web site is referred to in this work as a citation and/or a potential source of further information does not mean that the author or the publisher endorses the information the organization or Web site may provide or recommendations it may make. Further, readers should be aware that Internet Web sites listed in this work may have changed or disappeared between when this work was written and when it is read.

Printed in the United States
BOOK PRODUCTION DESIGN: T.L. Price • design@tlpricefreelance.com

Baldwinsville Public Library
East Tennessee Street
Baldwinsville, NY 027-2575

WITHDRAWN

Reduce. Reuse.
RECYCLE.

A decade ago, Atlantic Publishing signed the Green Press Initiative. These guidelines promote environmentally friendly practices, such as using recycled stock and vegetable-based inks, avoiding waste, choosing energy-efficient resources, and promoting a no-pulping policy. We now use 100-percent recycled stock on all our books. The results: in one year, switching to post-consumer recycled stock saved 24 mature trees, 5,000 gallons of water, the equivalent of the total energy used for one home in a year, and the equivalent of the greenhouse gases from one car driven for a year.

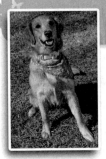 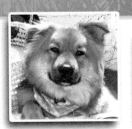 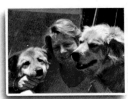

Over the years, we have adopted a number of dogs from rescues and shelters. First there was Bear and after he passed, Ginger and Scout. Now, we have Kira, another rescue. They have brought immense joy and love not just into our lives, but into the lives of all who met them.

We want you to know a portion of the profits of this book will be donated in Bear, Ginger and Scout's memory to local animal shelters, parks, conservation organizations, and other individuals and nonprofit organizations in need of assistance.

– *Douglas & Sherri Brown*,
President & Vice-President of Atlantic Publishing

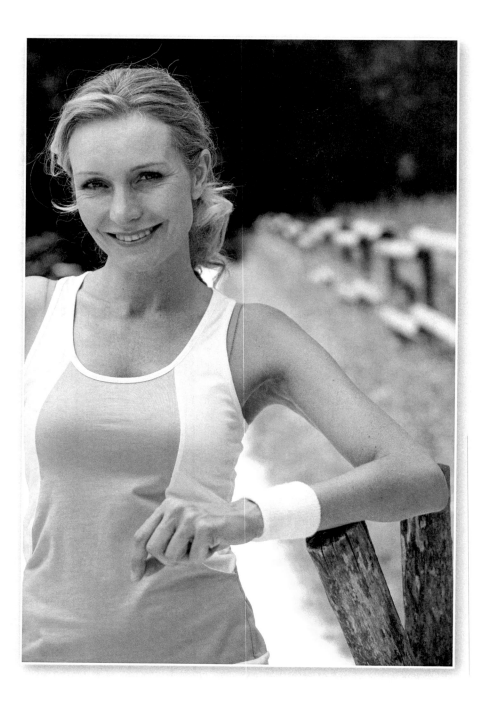

Table of Contents

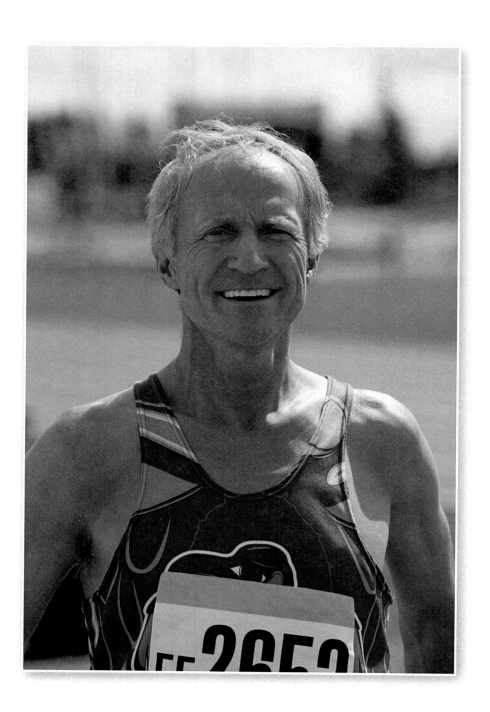

DEDICATIONS

Susan Petrosky Cotler

Mitchell and Amanda Cotler

Dr. Phillip Marone M.D. and Dr. Michael Schaefer M.D.
Both inspired me through their sports medicine approach for
the Phillies and Cubs in my career in orthopedic surgery.

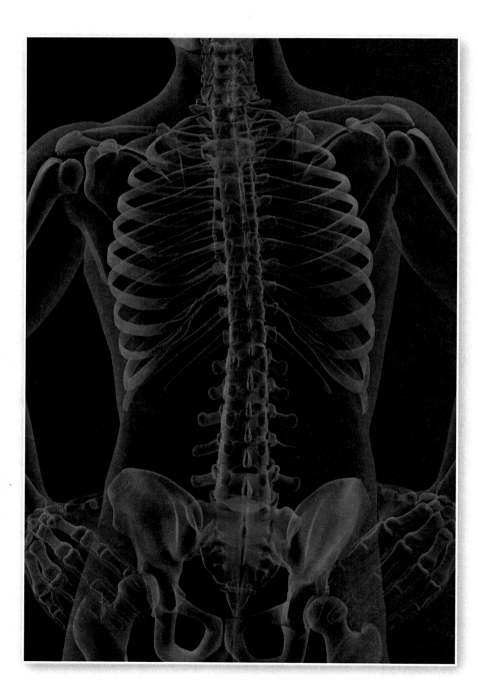

Author Bio

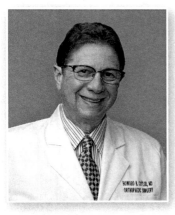

Howard B. Cotler, M.D., FACS, FAAOS is board certified and recertified in Orthopedic Surgery. He is a fellow of the American Academy of Orthopedic Surgery and the American College of Surgeons. He received his medical degree in 1979 from Jefferson Medical College of Thomas Jefferson University in Philadelphia. In 1980, Dr. Cotler completed his surgical internship at Grady Memorial Hospital/Emory University in Atlanta. In 1984, he completed his orthopedic residency at Thomas Jefferson University Hospital.

Dr. Cotler subsequently pursued advanced training in spine through two fellowships: one in acute spinal cord injury surgery with Northwestern University in Chicago in 1984 and another in Orthopedic Traumatology from Harborview Medical Center/University of Washington in Seattle in 1985. From 1985 to 1990, Dr. Cotler had both a clinical practice and an academic appointment at the University of Texas Medical School in Houston. In 1990, he became a founding partner and medical director for the Texas Back Institute of Houston. He was clinical associate professor of Orthopedic Surgery at the University of Texas

Medical School in Houston. In 1995 Dr. Cotler founded Gulf Coast Spine Care Limited PA.

If you like this book, you can find more information at **www.gulfcoastspinecare.com** and follow Dr. Cotler on Twitter, LinkedIn and Facebook.

Introduction

In this digital age, everyone wants faster. Faster smartphones, faster computers, faster cars, faster Internet, and even faster recovery from injury and surgery. So in this fast-paced world, how should you to recover your body after some type of insult or surgery? After all you have the same old body, which is only getting older every day. How can you restore some form of youth for accelerated recovery? How can you return to activities (work, school, family, hobbies, sports) faster than previous generations with the least inconvenience and cost?

The idea of accelerated recovery comes from professor Henrique Kehlet, a Danish surgeon who in the early 90s developed a program to speed up recovery after colorectal surgery. Now total joint replacement, spine surgery and trauma surgery have also seen the benefits of this type of approach.

All patients may want accelerated recovery, but how does the science and practice of medicine support the goal? We must be realistic about what is possible and not be enticed by false hopes. Although unsupported science may be very appealing, if it is ineffective then it may be purely a drain on your wallet.

As a board-certified orthopedic surgeon who is subspecialized in spine care, I hope to share my 30 years of experience to help with decision-making. After all, without the experience of previous generations we probably would not be where we are today. My personal background as an orthopedic trauma surgeon focused on stabilizing all traumatic injuries for the polytrauma patient so they could recover after terrible injuries. But now with newer techniques we are able to apply minimally invasive techniques combined with additional services to decrease complications and length of hospital stay as well as result in faster recovery.

Through this book I hope that I am able to educate, enlighten and engage readers to make better choices toward their health goals and those of their family.

CHAPTER 1

The Station in Life

Life is a continuum of time and experiences. We are born, we grow and we experience, all the while our bodies continue to change and develop. But there comes a time when development stops and we begin to deteriorate. This deterioration is called aging. When this occurs, we must recognize exactly where we are at that stage in our life and understand the reality. This is necessary to meet proper expectations. A perfect example of the situation is a professional athlete who sustains a significant injury. Some athletes can recover both their health and abilities, while others can recover only their health and are unable to recover the abilities that allowed them to be a professional athlete. Thus, reality, injury, Father Time and the ability of the body to recover are important factors in realistic decision-making in regards to your health after injury.

Determining the station in life is important for setting proper expectations. First, one must determine if an injury is salvageable. Are the treatments to be palliative, curative, or somewhere in between? It is difficult to make predictions at first glance. Often an injury requires an evaluation, a tentative treatment plan and then modifications as the situation evolves.

After an injury, it is often possible to restore an ability as it was at the patient's station in life, but not to go back in time to an earlier state of being. Thus managing expectations is important when determining the outcome of your recovery.

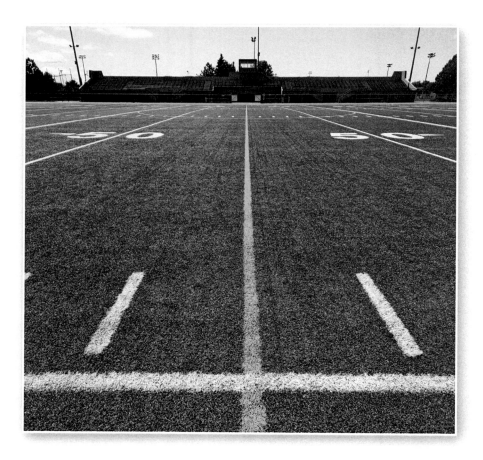

DALLAS COWBOY QUARTERBACKS:
Troy Aikman & Tony Romo

Troy Aikman is a Pro Football Hall of Fame quarterback who led the Dallas Cowboys to three Super Bowl wins during his 11-year tenure in the NFL. When Aikman retired at the age of 34, the commonly held belief was that multiple concussions led him to end his career earlier than he wanted-ed. But in 2013, Aikman himself admitted it was painful back spasms that caused him to leave the game.

Aikman underwent back surgery when he was 26, following his first Super Bowl victory. He recovered quickly and led his team to two more championships over the next six years. However, the wear he put on his body had a cumulative effect and by the time he was 34, he was being treated for back pain with regular epidural injections.

It was in a game against the Jacksonville Jaguars, when Tony Brackens tackled Aikman and slammed him on his back, that the superstar quarter-back immediately felt painful back spasm begin. Aikman was treated with additional shots the following week, but was unable to return to a pain-free state. At that point, Aikman knew his playing days were done.

This will prove relevant for current Dallas Cowboy quarterback Tony Romo because, at the time of his retirement, Aikman was the same age Romo was in 2013 when he underwent two back surgeries in less than eight months. The first operation was a procedure to remove a cyst from Romo's spine, with a second surgery the following December to repair a herniated disk.

Since 2013, Romo has been managing his recovery through stretching exercises — and at times injections — prior to or after practices and games.

He has also been working his abdominal and oblique muscles in order to enhance his rotational strength. However, even with rest and rehabilitation, an injury at that age can be career ending. Aikman said, "I'd get hit and there was no way to move. It severely limited me and how I was able to move around. We saw that with Tony the first two or three games of the season. He wasn't avoiding sacks and hits like he normally would."

Just two years later, in 2015, Romo suffered a broken collarbone early in the season that caused him to miss several games. After struggling upon his return, he reinjured his collarbone in late November and missed the rest of the season. While the injury is unrelated to his back issues from 2013, if he is experiencing the same lack of mobility that Aikman described, this could be contributing to ongoing health issues for Romo.

What Aikman describes he felt prior to his retirement and what Romo is currently enduring both demonstrate how age and high levels of physical demands can negatively impact recovery, even when rest and rehab are incorporated.

CHAPTER

2

The Science Of Aging

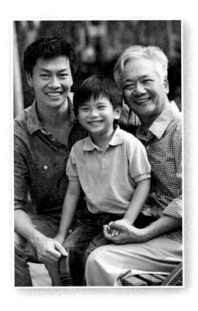

Aging is the process of change that occurs in a human being over time. Aging can refer to the cells within an organism or the organism itself. The causes of aging are unknown, but it is probably a combination of external and internal factors. While all humans age, there are some cells such as cancer cells, stem cells and germ cells which may live forever. Thus, the concept of immortality is present in spite of human cells only being able to survive 50 cell divisions.

THEORIES OF AGING

There are currently two theories regarding biological aging; the programmed aging theory and the damage theory. In the programmed aging theory, aging follows a timetable of growth, development, maintenance, repair and defense. In the damage theory, the environment bombards the organism and the cumulative damage causes aging. Regardless of how exactly our cells age, there are four pathways that influence the rate of aging, and these four pathways may be targeted to increase lifespan of the cell and organism.

The four main pathways that influence aging are:

1. Caloric restriction
2. Insulin/IGF-1 signaling pathway
3. Mitochondria electron transport chain
4. FOXO3/Sirtuin pathway

One of the current theories about aging is based on a protective mechanism called cell senescence. When a cell is damaged it either dies in a process called apoptosis, or it simply stops dividing. When a cell stops dividing it is called cell senescence. It has recently been learned that when cells opt to senesce they do not die. These cells keep aging, all the while secreting inflammatory cytokines (a type of protein). These cells produce a low level of chronic inflammation throughout the body with no obvious pathogen. It is believed that this process may be the main driver of aging. Focusing on this cell senesce may be a key to the evaluation and treatment of inflammation. This may be where the idea of the cranky old man/woman came from seeing as, as we age, we are in a constant state of inflammation.

SHRINKING

As we get older we have a tendency to shrink. Oftentimes this happens without us even noticing. Why does this happen and what effect does it have?

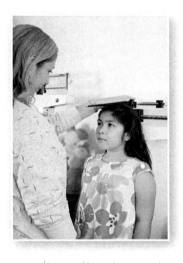

When a baby is born, the pediatrician measures the child on a monthly basis to determine the child's ability to thrive. Babies progress from a supine position, to crawling, to toddling, to walking, to jogging and then to running.

Starting at around 40 years of age, people tend to lose about 4/10 of an inch in height every decade. Some loss of height is a result of the normal aging process, and some loss of height may be related to disease. Men lose an average of 1.2 inches between the ages of 30–70, and 2 inches by age 80. Women lose an average of 2 inches between 30–70 and 3.1 inches by the age of 80.

Smoking cigarettes, drinking alcohol or caffeine excessively, extreme dieting, and taking steroids and other medications can accelerate height loss. Gravity plays a large role as well. As we get older we lose the water content inside our discs that separate the vertebral bodies of the spine. This loss of hydration results in a drying out and collapse of the discs. Fractures due to soft bone or osteoporosis can result in a spinal deformity known as kyphosis, which is an extreme rounding of the back. Loss of abdominal muscle tone results in increased spinal deformity. One's height is the greatest in the morning after sleeping and allowing the discs to rehydrate overnight. After being up and active all day water shifts out of the discs and they have a tendency to contract resulting in increased height loss in the evening compared to the morning.

Accelerated height loss is a marker of high risk for hip fractures in women and heart disease in men. Women have a tendency to display their height loss more obviously due to their lower muscle mass compared to men. It should be noted that approximately 20 percent of people do not shrink primarily due to a combination of genetics and following healthy habits throughout their lives.

Three major ways to dramatically reduce shrinking include:

1. Feeding your bones by treating osteopenia/osteoporosis
2. Exercising
3. Stopping smoking

CHAPTER 3

The Science Of Injury

Injury is defined as damage to the body. An injury may be classified by cause, modality, location or activity. Following an injury, the body stimulates the neuroendocrine system and the inflammatory response is initiated. Additionally there is damage to blood vessels, which initiates the clotting cascade. This process helps to maintain a healthy blood pressure and stimulate a healing response.

ACUTE/SUBACUTE STAGE

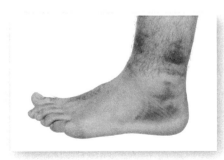

With an injury, the body feels a sharp swelling, warmth, redness, altered function and pain. In an acute, or sudden, injury the body generates an inflammatory response that lasts 48–72 hours. The body must stop bleeding and wall off the injured area. Inflammation is necessary to bring different cells and chemical mediators for clot formation, but too much inflammation results in severe edema (swelling), which may further injure the surrounding tissues. At the end of acute inflammation, a stage of passive congestion begins, which results in a normal level of swelling for the injury. This subacute phase begins at approximately 72 hours when acute inflammation stops.

CHRONIC STAGE

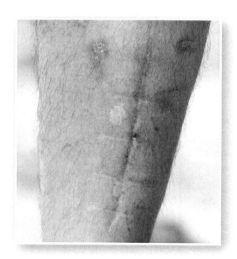

The chronic stage of injury is divided into the tissue healing phase and the maturation, or remodeling, phase. The tissue-healing phase lasts from seven to 14 days while the remodeling stage lasts for approximately one year. A condition becomes chronic if an acute inflammatory process continues due to either re-injury or chronic irritation. In the tissue-healing phase, scar tissue begins to form through the development of granulation tissue, which is new connective tissue. At three weeks the scar begins to form. If inflammation continues during scar formation, there are chances developing adhesive capsulitis (the freezing of joints) due to tissue damage to muscle, ligaments and tendons. The final stage is one of remodeling with maturation. In this remodeling phase, the collagen begins to realign in the scar based upon tensile stress. This strengthening of the scar may take years.

STAGES OF INJURY	
Acute (first 72 hours)	acute inflammatory stage
Subacute (one week)	passive congestion
Chronic (over two weeks)	fibroblastic repair + maturation-remodeling

Can your body heal itself? Generally the body is a wonderfully equipped natural self repair mechanism. With a positive mindset, excellent nutrition, rest and protection of your body, the body is able to very nicely recover from illness or injury.

Here are some simple steps to activate your bodies self repair mechanisms:

> Believe you can heal yourself
> Find the right support
> Listen to your body and your intuition
> Diagnose the causes of your illness
> Write the prescription for yourself
> Surrender your attachment to outcomes

If you have done all of the above and still notice no improvement, do not be stubborn and continue to wish and hope for a good outcome. Consult a doctor or get a second opinion if necessary.

STRUCTURAL INJURY

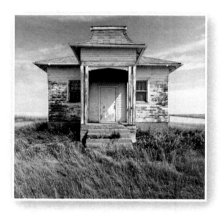

Injuries can be divided into either soft-tissue and/or bone/structural injury. Think of a house where the foundation represents structural integrity and the house represents the soft-tissue or wrapping. When paint and plaster are peeling in the house, this may represent a cosmetic problem or a structural problem. If it is just wear and tear of the exterior, then some cosmetic work involving paint and plaster are in order. A house that has a foundation problem represents a real challenge to the owner. A foundation is the building block of the house. So in a house that has foundation problems, just doing cosmetic work or a patch job will not cure the problem, and painting and plaster will only hide the problem for a while.

A broken leg is a painful condition. When a leg is broken it is often obvious. So the question is would you continue to run on the broken leg? Or would you take pain medications to mask the pain and then run on it?

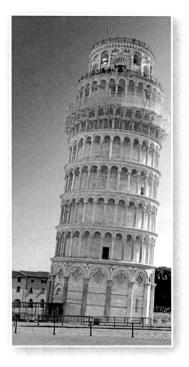

The point of these examples is when there is a structural problem, it often requires a structural solution. The deformed leg is not structurally sound to walk on and taking narcotics to deaden the pain so you can walk on it will only increase injury to the limb. The broken leg needs to be fixed so you can return back to an active lifestyle. The correction requires surgery. Not performing the surgery will result in deformity, loss of abilities, chronic pain and possibly loss of limb. By repairing the bone or structural abnormality, oftentimes the soft-tissue will improve on its own with natural healing.

The same analogy holds true with your body. If the foundation is damaged then it will have difficulty bearing weight and this will either result in pain or deformity. This is why when you see people who complain of back pain oftentimes they are tilted or cannot straighten up. This is a structural problem similar to your house foundation. Structural problems generally require structural solutions. Performing Band-Aid solutions on structural problems is doomed to failure.

THE RISKS OF A SEDENTARY LIFESTYLE

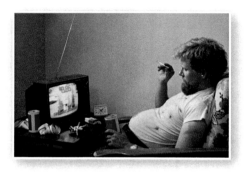
For those who choose or are forced into a sedentary lifestyle, the chance of death significantly increases. Although the pain from an injury may cause you to lead a sedentary lifestyle, it is important that you keep active.

The facts are:

> ➤ Inactivity increases with age
> ➤ Women are more likely to be sedentary than men
> ➤ Non-Hispanic white males are more likely to engage in physical activity than Hispanic or non-Hispanic black males

Less active less fit people have a greater risk of developing:

> ➤ Hypertension
> ➤ Heart disease
> ➤ Anxiety and depression
> ➤ Cancer
> ➤ Diabetes
> ➤ High cholesterol

It should also be recognized that patients with chronic disease, paralysis and cancer are also subjected to the same additional risks as those who elect to be inactive.

GETTING ACTIVE

Weight loss is important to decrease the load carried by your joints. Take for example your knees, which carry four times your body weight. If you weigh 180 pounds the normal pressure on your knees is 720 pounds. Say you then lose 20 pounds. Then the pressure on your knees drops down to 640. Ideally you should keep your weight a healthy range with a BMI (body mass index) of 18.5 to 24.9.

Protecting your joints can help you control your daily arthritis joint pain. When standing or walking, do not stand too long in one place, keep your feet wide apart to distribute your weight evenly, and ditch the high heels. When sitting or resting, change positions frequently. When performing material handling, lift objects with your legs, and avoid excessive squatting or kneeling.

Whether it is a hip joint, a knee joint, a finger joint, or a spine joint, the principles are the same. The only difference with spine joints is that there are more risks inherent, as one must have concerns for protecting the spinal cord and nerve roots; they are not replaceable and result in significant impairment when damaged.

With inactivity or after any surgery there is the potential for risks or complications. Two of the most serious complications that can occur after spine surgery involve blood clots. When blood clots develop inside the veins of the legs it is known as deep venous thrombosis (DVT). Blood clots may form in the large veins of the calf or the veins of the thigh. These clots can subsequently extend into the veins of the pelvis and should they become dislodged and travel to the lung, they become pulmonary emboli (PE). Once the clot arrives in the lung it obstructs tiny vessels and cuts off the blood supply to that portion of the lung. The lung subsequently collapses and breathing is impaired.

The risk of developing a blood clot is much higher following surgery involving the lower extremities. But certainly people who have been in severe pain and have had limited ability to walk are also more likely to develop blood clots than someone who is active.

Two ways to prevent these clots are:

1. Mechanical – elastic stockings and pulsatile compression devices
2. Medical – using blood thinners

Blood that is moving is less likely to clot, so moving is important to preventing blood clots. Pumping your feet up and down, isometric muscle contraction of your legs and walking as soon as possible after surgery are usually effective.

After surgery, the body tries to stop bleeding associated with the surgery and forms a blood clot. In addition, injury to blood vessels surrounding the surgical site from normal retraction can also set off the clotting process. Blood that becomes stagnant also tends to clot. A blood clot that forms and compresses the spinal cord or nerve is known as an epidural hematoma. These hematomas may require evacuation if a neurologic problem begins to develop.

The Science of Post-Injury Recovery

Most acute injuries may be treated at home following the RICE principle. RICE stands for:

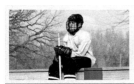 **R**est and immobilization

 Ice

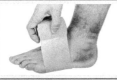 **C**ompression

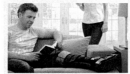 **E**levation

For the first 48–72 hours after injury, RICE is immediately applied. The goal during this period of time is to prevent further injury, decrease the amount of swelling and reduce pain. In order to decrease the amount of time in recovery, it is imperative to decrease the swelling.

REST

The first thing to do is protect the injured area from further damage. Once an injury occurs, you must immediately stop whatever you are doing. Next, stop using the injured area by getting into a position of comfort, using mobility aids (crutches, walker, wheelchair), or wearing a splint or brace. By using these techniques you help prevent further injury. Continued insult to the injury will cause increased circulation to the injured area, increased bleeding, increased swelling and possibly further damage to the surrounding muscle.

ICE

Ice or cryotherapy can be used to stop bleeding by causing constriction of local tissue and vessels. Ice also causes a numbing effect to the local area and is a very effective pain reliever.

COMPRESSION

After the ice is removed, a light compression wrap may be applied. This wrap may be applied to the injured area to control swelling. We know that continued ongoing swelling will delay healing of the injured area.

Compression devices may take the form of elastic or ace bandages, elastic sleeves for extremities, or a lumbar support for the low back. Be careful when applying an elastic wrap such as an Ace bandage; you do not want it to create a tourniquet effect, as this will impair circulation.

ELEVATION

The last principle of RICE is elevation. An injured limb should be elevated above the heart in order to reduce the blood flow to the injured area and minimize the swelling. This way the injured may return to activity or play quickly.

After a day or two of RICE treatment, symptoms usually begin to resolve. Should symptoms be severe or not begin to resolve as expected a visit to the emergency room or physician is recommended.

Once the healing process has begun, light massage or low-level laser therapy (LLLT) may be used to improve tissue healing after all swelling has resolved. Gentle range of motion or stretching may also be performed to improve healing tissue. Heat may be used to increase blood flow and promote healing once the injury has progressed out of the acute phase.

MOVEMENT AFTER INJURY

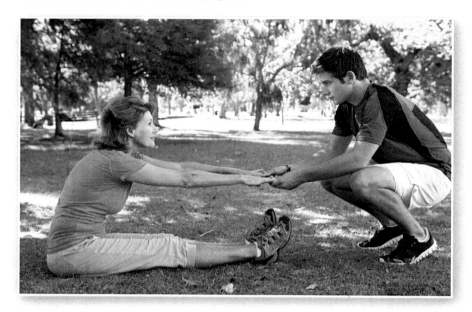

A certain amount of inflammation is essential for tissue healing. It has been found that the inflammatory cells produce IGF-1 (insulin-like growth factor-1), which is a hormone that increases the rate of muscle regeneration and heals damaged tissues. In a low oxygen area, IGF-1 promotes muscle cell division, which results in an atrophy of muscles similar to that of aging. Thus, in order to achieve maximal recovery, an oxygen-rich environment needs to be present so IGF-1 may continue to promote muscle cell differentiation.

In order to recover one's former self there is a process whereby milestones are achieved and progress continues.

The process of recovery:

1. Healing of tissues
2. Restore full range of motion
3. Restore function
4. Restore fluidity (gait)
5. Regain muscle strength
6. Regain endurance
7. Regain skills
8. Regain confidence

Whether it is a sports injury, workers' compensation injury, or just a recovery from a spontaneous occurrence, this process should be understood and followed to prevent flare-ups resulting in setbacks.

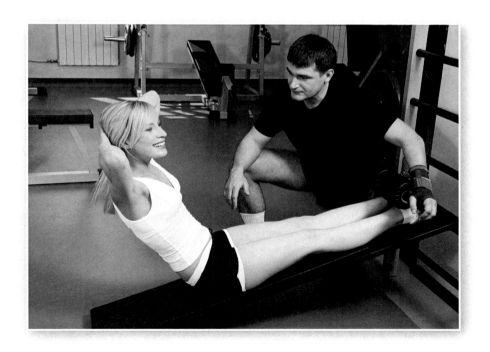

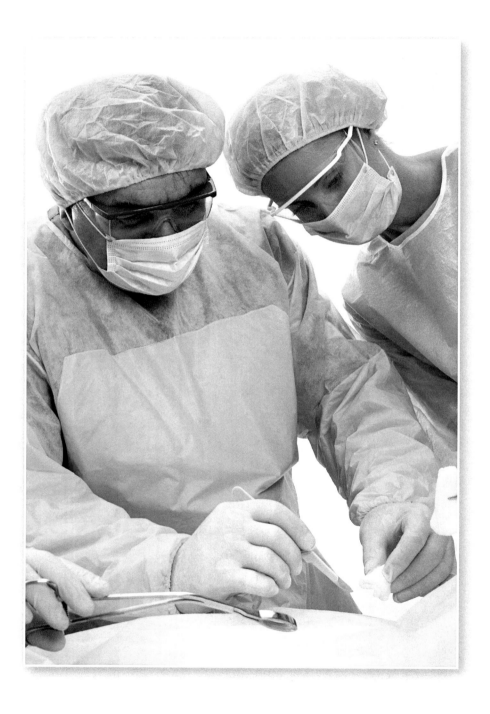

CHAPTER 5

The Science of Post Surgery Recovery

Just as the German autobahn is fast moving, so is life. The necessity of surgery already puts a damper on your life, so it makes sense that you would like to spend the least amount of time away from activities during recovery, with the least inconvenience and cost. A Danish surgeon, professor Henrique Kehlet developed a program in the early 90s to speed up recovery from colorectal surgery. We have taken these principles and applied it to musculoskeletal disorders requiring surgery. Total joint replacement, spine surgery, trauma surgery and surgery of sports injuries need the most assistance for accelerated recovery.

Ever hear your grandmother say "A stitch in time saves nine"? The intent of the statement is to say "Don't procrastinate!" In general conversation the phrase "A stitch in time saves nine" means to spend a little time now performing a task in order to prevent a larger task later. This essentially means it is better do deal with the smaller problem now than a larger problem later. Sometimes similar situations occur when dealing with painful musculoskeletal conditions.

Most people do not want to have surgery. It is natural for people to wish and hope that their condition is self-limiting and will resolve itself relatively quickly. There are occasions when procrastination can result in a worsening of the condition and make correction more difficult. If someone finds themselves in this situation it is important to be educated about the problem, find a physician you feel comfortable with and consider a second opinion. Prompt decisions can prevent irreversible damage.

In order to learn how to make the correct decision regarding surgery, you need to learn how to synthesize an overwhelming amount of incoming information and to make the best decision in a timely fashion. The best way to take a volume of information, synthesize it and make a decision is to learn how to deal with the hierarchy of knowledge.

Hierarchy of knowledge:

1. Gut instincts
2. Data
3. Information
4. Knowledge

When it comes time to make a big life decision, such as having surgery, consider the following seven steps of making a decision without regret:

1. Have a life vision
2. Evaluate the pros and cons
3. Discuss with a friend
4. Invoke a higher power
5. Flip a coin, but decide what you would choose before the flip
6. Ask questions
7. Don't regret

ACCELERATED RECOVERY PROGRAM

Orthopedic surgeries are performed to reduce pain, improve function and correct deformity. The Accelerated Postoperative Recovery (APR) is a program developed for the patient who requires orthopedic surgery to return to an active productive life.

The program:

➤ Allows you and your surgeon to develop a partnership for your recovery
➤ Decreases your time in the hospital
➤ Saves you money
➤ Increases your comfort
➤ Maximizes your recovery
➤ Decreases dehydration and starvation
➤ Lowers body reaction to stress
➤ Avoids complications

In order to return you back to health as soon as possible after your operation, it is important to get you out of bed, walking, eating and drinking, and off of prescribed narcotics as soon as possible. Essentially we are talking about returning you back to a normal life as soon as possible, considering the injury, required treatment and your stage in life. By speeding up the recuperation process, you will be less likely to experience complications such as:

- ➤ Wound infections
- ➤ Abdominal problems – nausea, vomiting, constipation, obstruction
- ➤ Blood clots – legs, lungs, wound
- ➤ Pneumonia
- ➤ Need for additional surgery

In order to have a successful outcome it is important that you take an active role in your recovery.

Before surgery, go through the following checklist.

1. Educate yourself about the cause of your problem
2. Review your options of care
3. Schedule a preoperative medical evaluation
4. Schedule a preoperative anesthesia evaluation
5. Review hospital laboratory studies
6. Maintain a healthy diet
7. Stop smoking
8. Lose weight, if necessary
9. Exercise your muscles and lungs
10. Decrease narcotics usage

11. Stop anti-inflammatories and blood thinners seven days before surgery

12. Stop herbals, supplements and over-the-counter medications

Before surgery

It is important that you remain active and take a walk every day. Also begin your breathing exercises.

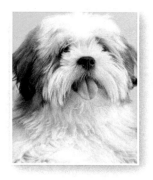

1. Pant like a puppy dog
2. Take a deep breath and hold it for five to 10 seconds. Repeat 10 times.
3. If are using an incentives spirometer, take a deep breath and hold it as you try to get the indicator to the goal position. Repeat 10 times.

These three things will keep your lungs in better shape before your surgery.

Five days before surgery

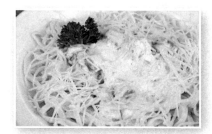

Maintain a normal diet, but add Nestlé Impact (Nestlé Health Science, Epalinges, Switzerland), a nutrition supplement used to prepare your body for surgery and accelerate your body's healing after surgery, to your routine. Drink the Impact with meals or between meals. Make sure you drink three 8-ounce cartons per day. If you are diabetic, monitor your sugar more carefully or drink 4 ounces of Impact six times a day. Impact has a vanilla flavor but you may wish to add 2 tablespoons of chocolate or strawberry flavoring to the Impact. It is best when served cold.

One to two days before surgery

Increase carbohydrates or carb load, with foods such as pasta, rice, cereals, bread, grains, fruits, beans and milk.

Eight hours before surgery

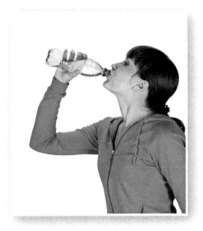

Be sure to stop all solid foods and drink 32 ounces (4 cups) of Powerade or Gatorade. You may drink clear liquids until four to six hours before your operation, but check with the anesthesiologist.

The night before surgery and the morning of surgery, take a hot shower with an antibacterial soap such as Hibiclens (Mölnlycke Health Care, Gothenburg, Sweden). The body should be cleansed from head to toe.

After surgery

The goals are to:

> Walk as soon as possible

> Begin clear liquids and advance as tolerated

> Avoid constipation (chew gum to aid digestion and G.I. motility)

> Maintain hydration and nutrition

> Carefully control your blood sugars (if diabetic)

> Take a daily shower for hygiene

Surgery is a major impact to your body — not only physically but also mentally. You have to recover from it. The Accelerated Postoperative Recovery (APR) program is designed to keep your body functioning as normal as possible in spite of having surgery.

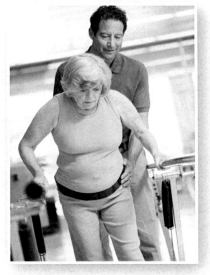

The above program is primarily for elective or scheduled surgery. In those cases requiring emergency surgery, the program must be modified. With the lack of preparation and/or the skipping of steps, the risk of complications increases.

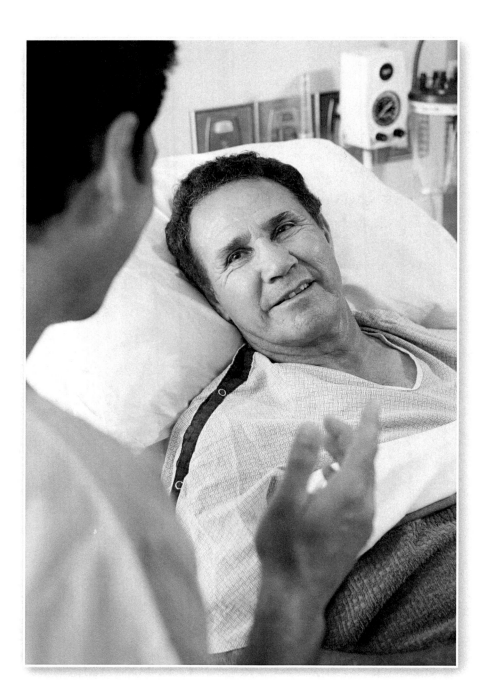

CHAPTER 6

Techniques For Accelerated Recovery

REST

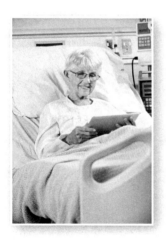

The idea of total bed rest as a treatment has been replaced with the concept of early mobilization or active rehabilitation. It has been found that the stimulation derived from movement is crucial to early healing after injury or surgery. Bed rest results in muscle atrophy, and muscle atrophy results in the loss of strength. This is what we call the **disease of inactivity**. With injury there is a rapid loss of muscle mass due to inactivity. **In fact, it takes three times the amount of time you were inactive to recover the muscle mass you lost during that period of inactivity.** So, add injury to inactivity and you have a prolonged period of dysfunction.

There comes a time when early mobilization or active rehabilitation must be tempered by avoiding placing excessive stress on an injury, which could result in severely fatigued muscles or additional damage to tissues. People have developed arbitrary techniques for getting over an injury by various forms of rest. Some prefer the overkill method where all activities are stopped for prolonged periods. Others try the minimal rest to stop the symptoms and then try to battle back. There are flaws with both ways of thinking.

Here are some helpful hints in deciding which method will work best for you.

> ➤ Decide how deep you want to bury the injury.
> ➤ Do not be afraid to test your recovery.
> ➤ Old problems are slow to go away and usually require more rest or a slower pace for rehabilitation.

Thus there is a need for a careful balance between protected healing and rehabilitation. Relapse sets the stage for prolonged periods of dysfunction.

CASE STUDY:
Tiger Woods

In October of 2015, Tiger Woods underwent a follow-up procedure to relieve discomfort in his back after undergoing microdiscectomy surgery just one month prior. This procedure was the third of three back operations in 21 months. In simple terms, the doctors removed a small disc fragment that was pinching a nerve in his back and causing him continued issues in regaining his status as one of the world's premier golf players.

In order to prepare for a return in early 2016, Woods planned to rest over the remainder of the 2015 schedule and off-season. As of October of 2015, Woods still reported feeling stiff and had yet to begin the rehab process. Two years earlier, he returned to play just three months after surgery and later admitted that he "tried to will himself through tournaments when it may have been best to remain outside the ropes."

Other golf players who experience similar surgeries have reported needing up to a year or longer to recover and be pain free. No stranger to the injury and recovery process, Woods might be feeling the impact of aging as he nears 40. Recognizing that he might need a longer period to heal, his mindset from his early surgeries seems to have changed, with him placing a stronger emphasis on recovery time and the process itself.

Woods will need to not only give his tissues time to heal, he will need to slowly rebuild his muscle strength and regain his full range of motion in order to get his golf swing back to where he is confident in his game again. The rest he is taking after his surgery will actually be paramount to expediting his recovery process and preventing further complications.

MOTION VERSUS IMMOBILIZATION

When someone breaks an arm, a splint is often applied to immobilize the arm so that the sharp bone fragments do not further damage the surrounding muscle. Once the bone is stabilized, early, protected motion may begin. In order to not overly stress the soft tissues, the use of an arm sling or splint/ cast to limit motion and protect the injured area may be necessary.

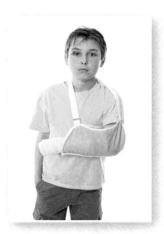

With any injury, we need to carefully balance the need to protect tissue with the need to move those same tissues in order to effect a faster and stronger healing process. Walking this tight rope is very challenging; one wrong move either way will be a setback on your path to recovery.

MEDICATIONS

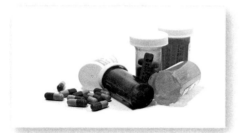

There are many medications that may be used in an accelerated recovery program. In recent years there has been a shift from narcotic pain medications to other medications that do not have the same risk profile as narcotics. Rampant abuse, overdose and the proliferation of psychiatric disease have necessitated this shift. We will present the medications for consideration.

PRESCRIPTION PAIN MEDICATIONS

Prescription medications come in the form of narcotics, muscle relaxers, corticosteroids, depressants and anti-seizure medications. They help modulate the sensation of pain.

Narcotic or opioid pain relievers should only be used for severe pain and for short periods of time. The use of narcotics for more than three to four weeks is not recommended. Narcotics block the feeling of pain and can result in abuse, dependency or addiction. Some prescription narcotics include:

> Codeine
> Fentanyl— available as a patch
> Hydrocodone
> Hydromorphone
> Morphine
> Oxycodone
> Tramadol

Muscle relaxers relax contracted muscles, but can be extremely sedating. We usually recommend that these be taken at bedtime in order to prevent spasms, prevent over sedation during the day and aid in a restful night's sleep. Some muscle relaxers include:

> Carisoprodol — may be more addictive than others
> Cyclobenzaprine
> Diazepam
> Methocarbamol

Antidepressants work by changing certain levels of chemicals in your brain and thus changing the way your brain notices pain. Generally, antidepressants are used for chronic pain situations, and include:

> Amitriptyline
> Desipramine
> Duloxetine
> Imipramine
> Nortriptyline

Anti-seizure and anticonvulsant medications are also effective for the treatment of pain. The following medications change the electric signals in your brain and work best for pain that is caused by nerve damage:

> Carbamazepine
> Gabapentin
> Lamotrigine
> Pregabalin
> Valproic acid

All of these drugs have their own side effects. Common side effects include weight gain or weight loss, loss of appetite, upset stomach, rashes, drowsiness or feelings of confusion and headaches. Do not take these drugs unless you are under a doctor's care. Do not stop these drugs suddenly or change dosage without discussing it with your physician.

Injectable pain medications should only be used as a last resort as there are greater chances for dependency and addiction. Overdose is a major concern.

The recent addition of intravenous Tylenol, Ofirmev (Mallinckrodt Pharmaceuticals, Dublin, Ireland) has been a new medication used for postoperative pain. Intravenous Tylenol has a fast onset of pain relieving action and also bypasses the liver, decreasing the potential for hepatic injury. The lack of adverse side effects offer a strong positive recommendation for intravenous Tylenol as compared to other pain relievers such as narcotics.

Lastly injectable forms of local anesthetic such as bupivacaine liposome, Exparel (Pacira Pharmaceuticals Inc., Parsippany, New Jersey) when injected into a postoperative area will afford approximately three days of delayed release of local anesthetics. It is given as a single injection dose with a high safety profile.

TOPICAL PAIN MEDICATIONS

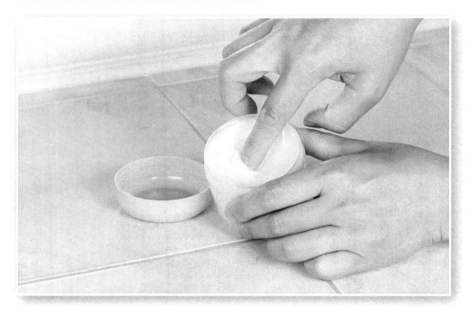

Topical pain medications are advantageous to decrease or avoid narcotic pain medications and give a feeling of pain relief without the side effects. Common topical pain medications include:

> ➤ Local anesthetics (lidocaine patches)
> ➤ Pain medications (anti-inflammatory drugs, narcotic pain relievers and topical pain relievers)
> ➤ Counterirritants (contain menthol, eucalyptus, or oil of wintergreen)

Do not use a topical pain reliever if the skin is not normal (such as an open wound or rash). Avoid applying too much as overdose is possible.

MEDICATIONS FOR INFLAMMATION

Medications used to manage inflammation of the musculoskeletal system either caused by arthritis or other disorders are usually categorized into either steroidal or nonsteroidal anti-inflammatory medications. The use of these medications can cause serious side effects including stomach ulcers and bleeding. Also these medications may be harmful when used with blood thinning medicines and alcohol.

Nonsteroidal anti-inflammatory drugs (NSAIDs) are used to manage pain and inflammation. Commonly used NSAIDs include aspirin, ibuprofen, naproxen, diclofenac and celecoxib. When a body part is inflamed, it secretes prostaglandins, which result in inflammation, pain, swelling and fever/warmth. NSAIDs block the specific enzyme used by the body to make prostaglandins, which helps relieve the symptoms.

Common side effects of NSAIDs include:

➤ Elevated liver enzymes
➤ Diarrhea
➤ Headache
➤ Dizziness
➤ Hypertension
➤ Salt and fluid retention
➤ Ulcers

A stronger type of anti-inflammatory medication is the oral steroid category. Oral steroids come in many forms but are usually ordered as a Medrol Dosepak. The dose pack starts with a high dose and then tapers down to a lower dose over the course of five to six days. When used on a short-term basis there are generally few complications. Side effects include stomach ulcers, weight gain, osteoporosis, avascular necrosis of the hip joints and others. It is advised that diabetics not use oral steroids as they may dramatically increase blood sugars. Patients with an active infection should also avoid steroid use.

Other types of medication

Herbal medications are derived from plants that are used medicinally to treat health problems. Many herbs are felt to decrease inflammation and help manage pain. Yet caution should be exercised as these herbs not only have the potential to help, but also may have the potential to harm through side effects, allergic reactions and interactions with others substances or medications.

Herbal pain relief medications:

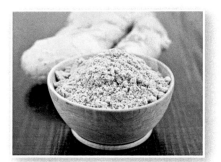

- ➤ Capsaicin
- ➤ Ginger
- ➤ Feverfew
- ➤ Turmeric
- ➤ Devil's claw

Herbs for pain management:

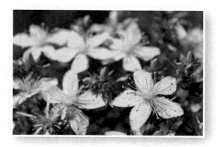

- ➤ Ginseng
- ➤ Kava kava
- ➤ St. John's Wort
- ➤ Valerian root

It should be noted that safety and efficacy research is still limited regarding the use of herbal therapies for pain management. The government does not regulate herbal products for quality. The best course of action is to talk to a health professional before testing out one of these herbal remedies. Certainly before any surgery, tell your physician and surgeon what you are taking and be prepared to stop two weeks prior to surgery.

Silver to fight infections

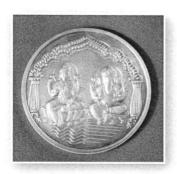

Silver and gold are best known as a currency for trade. Yet few know that the precious metal silver has also been used as a topical antimicrobial agent for hundreds of years. Silver wire had been placed in wounds, silver nitrate solutions have been used to cleanse wounds and silver antibiotic compounds have been used for burn therapy. Recently, wound dressings that contain elemental silver or silver releasing compounds have been developed. These dressings are easy to apply, provide sustained availability of silver, require less frequent dressing changes, manage fluids that can seep from wounds and facilitate the removal of dead tissue. Silver has been found to bind to bacterial cell membranes and cause bacterial cell death. It also has an anti-inflammatory effect, encouraging blood vessel formation and thus aiding in wound healing. It may be used in acute wounds or surgical incisions and chronic wounds.

Studies have found the use of silver dressings:

- ➤ Reduced time to wound healing
- ➤ Reduced dressing change frequency
- ➤ Shortened hospital stays
- ➤ Reduced need for pain medication
- ➤ Decreased methicillin resistant staphylococcus aureus (MRSA) bacteremia from infected wounds

This is just another example of old knowledge with new applications, resulting in safer modern healthcare.

HGH and IGF-1

Human growth hormone (HGH) and insulin-like growth factor-1 (IGF-1) have been known to boost muscle recovery, reduce fat and improve endurance. Growth hormone is synthesized in the pituitary gland and travels to the liver, which then responds by producing IGF-1. HGH has been used by professional athletes for many years due to its ability to increase the size of muscles. They have also recognized its benefit to accelerate recovery, but certifying professional associations have outlawed its use. IGF-1 has the ability to initiate the formation of bone and cartilage. The Food and Drug Administration (FDA) have approved the use of HGH for very specific indications of adult HGH deficiency, childhood idiopathic short stature and AIDS wasting syndrome.

Risks of taking human growth hormone include:

- ➤ Diabetes
- ➤ Hypertension
- ➤ Enlarged heart
- ➤ Muscle weakness
- ➤ Joint pain
- ➤ Fluid retention

Anabolic steroids

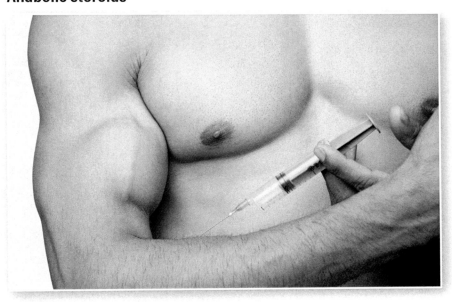

Anabolic androgen steroids or anabolic steroids have been taken by athletes to increase strength and muscle mass. The main anabolic steroid is testosterone, which is produced by the male body. Testosterone has two main effects — an anabolic effect, which promotes muscle building, and an androgenic effect, which gives facial hair and a deeper voice.

Anabolic steroids have been linked to helping athletes recover from a hard workout more quickly by reducing muscle damage.

The risks of taking anabolic steroids in men are:

- ➤ Impotence
- ➤ Infertility
- ➤ Prostate gland enlargement
- ➤ Baldness
- ➤ Prominent breasts
- ➤ Shrinking testicles

Women can develop:

- ➤ Baldness
- ➤ Period irregularity
- ➤ Increase in body hair

Both men and women can develop:

- ➤ Liver abnormalities and tumors
- ➤ Tendon rupture
- ➤ Acne
- ➤ Abnormal cholesterol
- ➤ Hypertension
- ➤ Cardiovascular problems
- ➤ Psychiatric illness
- ➤ Rage, aggressive behavior and violence
- ➤ Infections
- ➤ Inhibited development and growth

Erythropoietin

Erythropoietin (EPO) is a hormone used to treat anemia. By increasing the production of red blood cells and hemoglobin the movement of oxygen to muscles is improved. This increased oxygen helps fuel muscles. Endurance athletes, especially cyclists, have been known to use erythropoietin, also called blood doping. There are three types of blood doping; blood transfusions, use of erythropoietin (EPO) and injection of synthetic oxygen carriers (HBOCs and PFCs). The risks of its use include stroke, heart attack and pulmonary embolism.

Creatine

Creatine is a naturally occurring compound produced by your body that helps muscles to release energy. Creatine monohydrate is a supplement that may result in small gains in short-term bursts of power, yet there is no evidence that creatine enhances performance in aerobic or endurance sports. Possible side effects include stomach and muscle cramps, and weight gain. The use of high doses may result in liver and kidney damage.

Platelet-rich plasma (PRP)

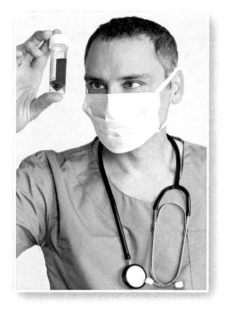

Platelet-rich plasma (PRP) has the potential to effectively treat tendon, ligament and muscle injuries. In blood there are two components — a liquid component called plasma and solid components called red cells, white cells and platelets. Platelets are important for clotting blood. In the platelets there are growth factors that are important for healing of injuries. Recently there have been good laboratory studies demonstrating increased concentration of growth factors in PRP, which can potentially accelerate the healing process. Human studies are ongoing. Nevertheless it is felt that PRP may be injected into an injured area or following surgery to accelerate the healing of damaged ligaments or muscle. The use of PRP for arthritis is still not defined.

Stem cell therapy

Stem cell therapy for musculoskeletal injury is *experimental.* Embryonic stem cells are pluripotent, meaning they can develop into any type of cell or tissue. Because of their plasticity and unlimited capacity for renewal, these are the most useful source of cells for transplantation. So far it is unknown whether stem cells will be of benefit for a patient's restoration of injured or worn-out body parts. A stem cell or pluripotent stem cell in an adult cell line possibly can give rise to every cell type in the body. Thus they represent a single source of cells that could be used to replace those that are damaged or diseased.

Most physicians would like to believe that if you aspirated bone marrow from the pelvis, centrifuge it to concentrate the adult stem cells, and then inject the stem cells into or around the damaged structure, the body would be able to restore or regenerate the damaged tissue. This concept for treatment has the greatest application for the restoration of degenerative discs. However, it is indeterminate whether embryonal or adult are the most effective for the pathology. Also, this procedure for harvesting of adult stem cells costs a few thousand dollars and is not covered by insurance.

For most of the stem cell studies there have been no control groups for comparison and, even without stem cell therapy, most low back pain often gets better with time. With longitudinal studies it has become evident that some treatments can become harmful. It is clearly too early to know if stem cell therapy is effective or safe.

PERFORMANCE-ENHANCING DRUGS

Athletes throughout history have sought the extra competitive edge. Some athletes have achieved this through equipment, innovative training and improved nutrition. Others have sought substances that alter their bodies to improve cognition and heighten their physical ability to achieve victory. Most athletes do not use performance-enhancing drugs but some choose victory at all cost.

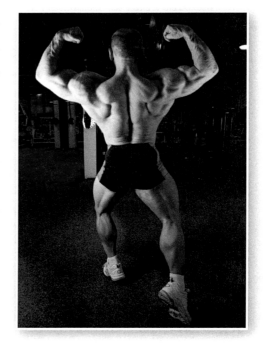

Our society has mimicked the athlete by consuming large volumes of caffeine, multivitamin supplements, protein shakes and creatine. In these unmonitored situations, increase risk to blood, liver and kidney function may be encountered. The use of testosterone supplements and human growth hormone has steadily increased among the lay public.

According to the World Anti-Doping Agency (WADA) the following substances are prohibited at all times:

1. Anabolic agents
2. Peptide hormones and growth hormones
3. Beta2-agonists
4. Hormone and metabolic modulators
5. Diuretics and masking agents

Non-athletes continue to be at the highest risk. Some of the risks placed on consumption result in a higher risk of infection, musculoskeletal problems causing tendon degeneration and rupture, premature closure of growth plates in the young athlete, and testicular atrophy, baldness and secondary acne due to decreased testosterone levels. There is a tremendous psychological facet, which may result in rage and psychosis. The most concerning are the cardiovascular effects, which may result in hypertension and arrhythmias.

On the playing field, clean play for all should be the mantra. In everyday life, healthy, safe life and longevity should be the mantra. One must remember that doping is fundamentally contrary to the spirit of sport and is an unhealthy way of trying to improve or recover body function.

CASE STUDY:
Cheating Olympians

In 2013, after years of allegations and denials, Lance Armstrong finally admitted to using performance-enhancing drugs. Prior to his admission, the U.S. Anti-Doping Agency released piles of evidence implicating Armstrong and his teammates in doping violations. He was stripped of his seven Tour de France titles and his Olympic bronze medal.

Armstrong was diagnosed and treated for testicular cancer in 1996. Over the following nine years, he won seven Tour de France competitions and faced heavy allegations of misconduct along the way. While Armstrong did need to take serious steps to recover from his fight against cancer in order to be able to return to competition, he proved that even recovering from a serious injury or illness needs to be done properly and legally.

Of course, the world of cycling is rich with doping violations and they are not all committed by individuals recovering from cancer battles. Floyd Landis, former Olympic athlete and long-time accuser of Armstrong, admitted in 2010 that he used performance-enhancing drugs most of his professional career as a road cyclist. Landis' statements were once considered damaging to the sport, but may have been the start of efforts to clean up cycling.

Cheating in sports through performance-enhancing drugs is not limited to cycling or even baseball, where it has been making headlines recently. Ben Johnson was a Canadian sprinter who was stripped of his gold medal from the 1988 Seoul Olympics where he set a new world record. But he wasn't alone — several of the eight finalists in that race tested positive or were later implicated in drug scandals.

Unfortunately, doping isn't even limited to male athletes. Marion Jones was a U.S. track and field competitor who won five medals (three gold) at the 2000 Sydney Olympics. In 2007, she admitted to lying to federal agents about her use of performance-enhancing drugs and pled guilty in court. She spent six months in jail and was stripped of her medals. The case that led to her conviction also implicated runners such as Kelli White and Regina Jacobs.

The World Anti-Doping Agency released a report in 2015 that showed a culture of doping has developed among athletes that compete in Olympic events worldwide. This certainly raises issues of fair play and what some athletes will do to gain a "competitive advantage." The negative health risks and odds for either immediate or eventual disgrace are not worth whatever short-term edge the athlete believes they are gaining.

TREATMENT MODALITIES

Ice and heat

Patients always ask physicians if they should use heat or ice on an injured or painful area of their body. As a general rule it is often recommended that ice be used for the first 24 hours of pain to decrease pain and swelling, but heat be used thereafter to increase circulatory flow and promote healing.

The facts are that there is some evidence that heat will decrease low back pain, but there is little proof that cold will help. Patients will need to decide which feels more beneficial to them.

How to use ice for low back pain:

> ➤ Use ice in a plastic bag covered by a towel, an ice pack, or a bag of frozen vegetables
> ➤ Ice area three times a day for approximately 20 minutes
> ➤ Ice after vigorous exercise or prolonged activity

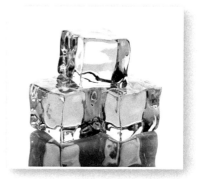

How to use heat for low back pain:

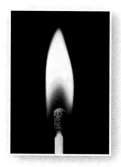

➤ Apply for 15 to 20 minutes at a time

➤ Moist heat is better than dry heat

➤ If using a heating pad, be careful to avoid burns

➤ Pharmacy heat wraps may also be beneficial

Try alternating:

➤ Use heat for 15 to 20 minutes, then ice for 10 to 15 minutes

These same techniques of ice and heat may be applied to an injury of the extremity. Be careful about falling asleep while applying ice or heat as serious burns/frostbite injuries have occurred.

Immersion therapy

Around the world, polar bear plunge events where people plunge into bodies of cold water, are held. Although these events are usually held for charity or even just for fun, some people do use this technique as a recovery method. Professional athletes have long used the ice bath or cold-water immersion during periods of intense exercise. This technique is controversial, potentially dangerous and has little scientific evidence to support its use. It has been speculated that the ice results in vasoconstriction and results in decreased swelling or inflammation.

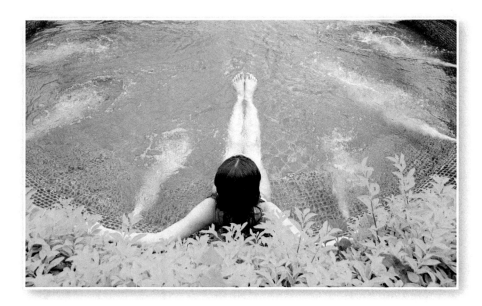

An American study found cold-water immersion has a slight effect on reducing soreness for up to 96 hours after exercise, lowers the levels of fatigue, and speeds up physical recovery. Yet a British study found no benefit for pain, swelling, isometric strength or function. The bottom line is that the truth is somewhere in between, where moderation is key. The use of ice before training can reduce the amount of lactic acid produced by muscles and speed up muscle recovery after exercise or injury.

A hot tub has several health advantages. The hot tub can reduce stress, ease muscle pain and improve circulation by dilating blood vessels. But remember, if a communal sauna is used there is the potential for the transmission of diseases such as Legionnaires' disease. There is also the possibility of contact dermatitis and cut cuticles from a manicure or pedicure becoming infected. Also, after a strenuous workout your inner core body temperature rises and immersion in hot water may cause dizziness, nausea, fatigue, heat exhaustion, heatstroke or even a heart attack. It is advisable to not use a hot tub for at least one hour or more after you stop working out. It is better to take a cool shower or bath, rehydrate and allow your body temperature to return back to normal with your breathing and heart rate.

TENS

Transcutaneous electrical nerve stimulation (TENS) uses electric current to stimulate nerves for therapeutic purposes. Electrical stimulation for pain has been known since 63 A.D. in ancient Rome. Benjamin Franklin was also a proponent of this method for pain relief. The modern TENS unit is credited to C. Norman Shealy.

The TENS unit is used as a noninvasive nerve stimulation for both acute and chronic pain. There is some evidence that is useful for pain, yet there is other evidence that does not support the use of TENS for chronic low back pain. Recent studies have suggested that patients with acute complete spinal cord injury may develop recovery of motor function with the use of transcutaneous electrical stimulation. It appears that the stimulation causes a reawakening of nerve connections.

Massage

Massage therapy involves working on the body with pressure, tension, mechanical aids, vibration or manually. The purpose of massage is to promote a feeling of well-being or relaxation. In a professional environment, the

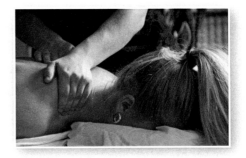

patient or client is treated either on a massage table, sitting in a massage chair or lying on a mat on the floor.

Evidence has been found that suggests massage was used in many ancient civilizations. In modern times, massage consumers spend approximately $4–6 billion on visits to massage therapists every year. Massage therapy has been particularly popular among amateur and professional athletes.

There are many types of massage therapies. Medical massage has involved techniques of tissue massage, myofascial release, trigger point therapy, osteopathic techniques, and craniosacral techniques. Medically, massage therapy has been found to reduce anxiety, blood pressure and heart rate. Massage therapy can also reduce pain, anxiety and depression.

Electric massage chair

Massage chairs have become popular as they can be used in the comfort of your own home. More people are beginning to recognize that the electric massage chair may symptomatically improve back pain, anxiety, depression and headaches. An electric massager can reduce or eliminate the discomfort caused by overused muscles, increase circulation and improve flexibility. Many of the electric massage chairs have a number of options including acupuncture pressure points, kneading, tapping, or rolling functions. Reflexology, different forms of massage including shiatsu, Swedish, deep, arm and leg stretch, and air compression may also be featured in certain models.

Electric massage chairs are expensive, but if you can afford it, they may represent a good investment for some symptomatic care.

Acupuncture

Acupuncture is a component of traditional Chinese medicine. Acupuncture is commonly used to treat pain. In acupuncture extremely thin needles are inserted through your skin at strategic points of your body.

Acupuncture is explained as a technique for balancing the flow of energy or life force, known as Chi. The Chi is believed to flow through pathways in your body. By inserting needles into specific points along these pathways, acupuncture therapists believe that your energy flow will rebalance.

Acupuncture is used for:

> Dental pain
> Fibromyalgia
> Headaches
> Neck pain
> Low back pain
> Osteoarthritis

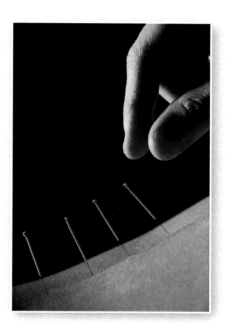

Risks are low but can include infection, organ injury, soreness and bruising, If you have a bleeding disorder, a pacemaker or are pregnant, then you are not a good candidate for acupuncture.

LLLT

Low-level laser therapy (LLLT), also known as cold laser therapy or photobiomodulation, is the application of light to promote tissue repair, reduce inflammation, induce analgesia or relieve pain. Think of a light going through a prism and all the colors of the rainbow coming out. In the electromagnetic spectrum light is made of various colors. The different colors represent wavelengths of light that are in a spectrum ranging from 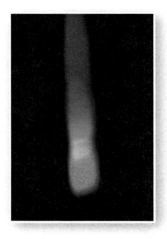 microwave to infrared to near infrared to visible light to ultraviolet to X-rays. Each laser of light has a different effect.

LLLT takes specific wavelengths of light and projects them through the skin to get specific effects. Think of LLLT like photosynthesis in plants. Just as sunshine is necessary for plants to grow and stay healthy, so can we use light for pain relief.

LLLT causes intracellular photochemical changes that lead to a cascade of downstream intracellular, extracellular and physiological changes. LLLT at low doses has been shown to enhance cell proliferation of fibroblasts, keratinocytes, endothelial cells and lymphocytes. This photostimulation of the mitochondria leads to activation of signaling pathways and increases regulation of transcription factors eventually giving rise to increased growth factors. LLLT can improve neovascularization, promote the development of new blood vessels and increase collagen synthesis to aid in the healing of acute and chronic wounds. Low doses of light have demonstrated the ability to heal skin, nerves, tendons, cartilage and bones. In addition, pain relief can be obtained by a nerve block without the use of xylocaine or numbing injection. These laser beams inhibit mitochondrial metabolism in C fibers and Delta fibers, reducing mitochondrial membrane potential and inducing a nerve blockade.

Acute orthopedic conditions such as strains, sprains, postsurgical pain, muscular neck and back pain, whiplash injury, radiculopathy and tendinitis are amenable to LLLT. Chronic conditions such as osteoarthritis, rheumatoid arthritis, frozen shoulder, epicondylitis (tennis elbow), carpal tunnel syndrome, tendinopathy, fibromyalgia, plantar fasciitis and complex regional pain syndromes may also benefit from LLLT.

There were 30 papers on LLLT published in 2012 and there have been over 300 clinical trials and 3,000 laboratory studies on LLLT. There are also several ongoing studies at Harvard. The device is FDA approved, approved in Europe and Canada and used by high-level amateur and professional athletes worldwide.

The four common clinical targets for LLLT are:

1. Site of injury to promote healing, remodeling and reduce inflammation
2. Lymph nodes to reduce swelling and inflammation
3. Induction of analgesia or pain relief
4. Trigger points to reduce tenderness and relax contracted muscles

The number of treatments required is dependent on several variables. The faster an injury is treated, the faster it resolves. But remember that if the treatment is started and not completed, oftentimes the pain returns worse than before, just like stopping antibiotics before an infection is cleared.

With this new technology patients can relieve pain and heal injuries without surgery, injections, pain medications or stomach ulcers. LLLT is beneficial for pain relief and can accelerate the body's ability to heal itself. LLLT should only be used as additional therapy for pain relief in patients with neuropathic pain and neurologic deficits. Lasers and LED do not correct situations involving structural deficits or instabilities whether in bone or soft-tissue.

Kinesiology taping

Kinesiology (kinesio) taping is the use of an elastic tape that may be applied to an injured part of the body. You see this quite often with athletes. This type of taping allows for range of motion. Kinesio tape may be used during an event, for rehabilitation, for alignment or for competition.

Kinesio tape is placed on the skin and pulls the upper layer of skin to create more space between the dermis and muscle. This creation of space is believed to relieve pressure on the lymphatic channels, therefore creating more available space for better lymphatic drainage. It is also thought that the taping provides a form of decompression to local sensory nerve fibers, which can become compressed during injury. Kinesio tape is also believed to affect deep muscles by allowing more room for the injured or swollen muscle. Additionally, kinesio taping can affect scars or contractures.

BRACES, WRAPS, SPLINTS AND CASTS

Back braces

A brace is a device that gives added physical support or strength to something. A brace used to immobilize the back may serve several functions. A brace may be an extra reminder to reinforce the idea of keeping the body in a specific position during activity. A brace may also be used to immobilize a part of the body to prevent motion.

Olympic weightlifters are probably some of the strongest athletes in the world. Their core muscles are strong and well conditioned. Yet you oftentimes see them performing with a weight belt. This weight belt is an extra reminder for them to prepare their core during their performance. Braces, which are used at the worksite, are designed with the idea of reminding the worker to prepare for a physical task and avoid injury.

Patients who have undergone a spine surgery or fusion often need a belt and suspenders approach to allow the area of their body to heal without excessive motion. When selecting a brace, a surgeon needs to account for four variables — the ability of the brace to be removed, the weight of the brace, the cost of the brace and lastly the counter forces applied by the brace. A brace that does not restrict motion is essentially just another piece of clothing.

Belly wraps and binders

What is a belly wrap? A belly wrap is a product that claims to aid people to lose abdominal weight faster during a workout. The claim is that the belly wrap heats up the midsection area during a workout, which is supposed to target weight loss in that area. There are claims that people have lost weight and decreased waist size by using these wraps.

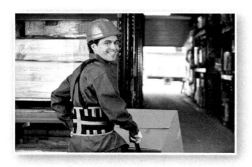

The reality is that weight loss is achieved not from losing fat but merely by fluid loss from excessive sweating. After the workout when one rehydrates the weight immediately returns. The danger of these bodysuits or body wraps is that excessive sweat can leave you susceptible to overheating, resulting in dizziness, weakness and mental confusion.

Alternatively, lumbar supports or binders are divided into lumbar supports and lumbosacral supports. The lumbar support provides support to the lumbar or low back area whereas the lumbosacral support provides support to both the lumbar and sacral or upper buttocks areas. For people who have an injury, illness or lack the ability to maintain proper posture on their own for longer periods of time, a binder is a good idea. For people who work in a job that require lifting or other strenuous exercise, a back binder can reduce the risk of back injury. Back binders should only be worn during periods of strenuous exercise or activities.

CASE STUDY:
Belly Binders

The American Council on Exercise states unequivocally that spot reduction is a myth, which means you cannot lose belly fat by using an apparatus to "tighten" your belly. Of course, it also means that you cannot flatten your stomach by only doing "crunch" exercises. You lose fat across your entire body by consuming fewer calories than you burn. Area specific exercises can build up specific muscle groups, but fat loss is overall, not spot reduction.

Therefore, belly wraps that have been popularized by reality television stars simply do not work. When pictures are published across the Internet of women in these devices, the benefits being seen are essentially that of a girdle. According to the Mayo Clinic, wearing a girdle-like contraption may improve appearance and posture, but it won't strengthen or tone your stomach muscles.

Due to the affects of compression, wearing a trimmer belt might create the illusion of weight loss because a waistline reduction may happen temporarily (which can be aided by water weight loss if the belt causes you to sweat and become dehydrated). However, studies have shown that your body will return to its normal shape and size soon after use.

Extremity wraps

Extremity wraps are useful to provide stability to an injury. The wrap is reported to take stress off of the joint and aid in the natural balance between joint and muscle strength. The feeling of security may be physical at first, but can develop into a psychological crutch.

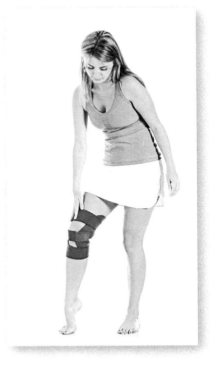

The main benefit of a wrap or sleeve seems to come from the heat retention that the sleeve provides. This translates into a feeling of joint warmth and thus results in less pain or discomfort of the joint while exercising. Knee sleeves appear to result in a better sense of joint positioning, which results in less fatigue. Knee sleeves are also helpful for managing pain in people who already have arthritis. It is important to note that compression has been found to only be helpful when worn for extended periods of time, not just for one or two hours while exercising.

NUTRITION

CALORIC REQUIREMENTS	
Female:	2,000–2,100 calories
Male:	2,700–2,900 calories
Athlete:	3,000–4,000 calories
Minor Surgery:	Increase caloric intake by 10–20 percent
Major Surgery:	Increase caloric intake by more than 20 percent

Most people are aware that good nutrition and a balanced diet are important for overall health. A balanced diet is one that gives your body the nutrition it needs to properly function. To be a truly balanced diet, the majority of your daily calories should

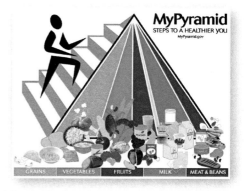

come from fresh fruits and vegetables, whole grains, and lean proteins. After an acute injury there is a period of traumatic shock and slow metabolism during the first few hours or days after injury. This phase is soon replaced by a period of fast metabolism that can last for weeks or months depending on the nature and extent of the injury, complications and obstacles to recovery. It is during this period of heightened metabolism that nutrition is most important.

Athletes need to consume more calories than the average person and that is because they require large amounts of energy. An athlete needs approximately 500 calories just to add muscle mass.

CASE STUDY:
Michael Phelps

Athletes might consume abnormally high levels of calories because they burn large amounts of energy during practice and competition. An athlete might need to expend up to 4,000 calories in a day as opposed to the 2,000 (for women) or 2,700 (for men) consumed by normal, active adults.

U.S. Olympic swimmer Michael Phelps told ESPN in 2008 that he regularly consumed between 8,000 and 10,000 calories in a day, and there was nothing "low carb" about his diet. He reported that pizza and pasta were a large part of his daily intake as well as fried egg sandwiches. However, even with all those carbs and high protein meals, it is unlikely that Phelps actually intakes that many calories by eating alone.

Having won 22 medals over three Olympic Games and competed as recently as the 2015 U.S. Winter National Championships, Phelps is still in prime physical condition. If you are thinking back to your parents' admonishment that you wait 30 minutes after a meal to swim, you are probably wondering when in the world Phelps would be able to practice if he spent his day eating that much food. The reality is that Phelps likely took supplements and formulated energy drinks in order to feed his caloric needs.

Remember though that when athletes leave their competitive sports, they often become heavy set if they do not change their dietary habits. An active adult might burn up to 700 calories in a run whereas Phelps is estimated to have burned up to 3,000 calories during a day of swim training. Once he stops operating at that level of activity, he will have to slow his caloric intake or risk becoming obese.

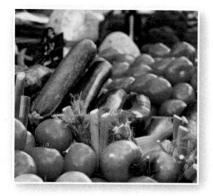 Having a healthy body includes preventing problems and healing injuries. The skeleton is surrounded by muscles and other structures that need good nutrition, including vitamins, to be strong enough to support the body and perform other functions.

The FDA does not evaluate supplements, so determining the need for supplements is left up to the consumer. In addition to managing inflammation and eating enough calories, supplementing with micronutrients and amino acids may help speed up the injury recovery process. One or two multivitamins per day seems to be important for the injured. Stresstabs do not appear to add any additional benefit.

The role of vitamins or nutrients:

> **Vitamin A** – For the immune system, tissue repair and bone formation. Typically 10,000 IU daily is recommended for a short period of time following serious injury

> **Vitamin B12** – For bone marrow. Four to seven mcg per day is recommended.

> **Vitamin C** – For collagen development, which allows tissue to heal.

> **Vitamin D** – Develops strong and healthy bones.

➤ **Vitamin K** – Helps bone stay strong and healthy, 120 mcg per day for an adult male, 90 mcg per day for an adult female, 15–100 mcg per day for children and adolescents.

➤ **Iron** – Needed for hemoglobin and myoglobin transport. Mostly available in diet and should only be supplemented if anemia is diagnosed.

➤ **Magnesium** – Important for muscle function and bone density. Most magnesium is absorbed from diet but those with kidney disease, Crohn's disease, parathyroid problems, taking medications for infection/diabetes/cancer, alcohol abusers, older adults, or those taking proton pump inhibitors for acid reflux may become deficient.

➤ **Calcium** – Essential for bone health.

Vitamin C

L-ascorbic acid (vitamin C) is an essential micronutrient used in multiple metabolic pathways. It also plays a key role in inflammation, protein metabolism, nerve function and the healing of tissues. Humans are unable to synthesize this essential vitamin and require intake from diet or supplements.

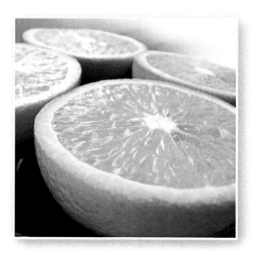

Vitamin C is found in many fruits and vegetables and is a common fortification in cereals, juices and multivitamins. The usual dietary dose for an adult is 100 mg/day, which is almost completely absorbed. The daily recommended intake for women is 75 mg and 90 mg for men. Smokers should consume an additional 35 mg per day due to the oxidative stress from cigarette smoke. Intake of 1,000 mg/day results in approximately 50 percent absorption. In high doses, vitamin C has a low toxicity.

Vitamin C is essential for:

> Fracture healing and prevention
> Bone mineral density
> Osteoarthritis prevention
> Complex regional pain

In a patient with a recent injury or requiring surgery, 500 mg of vitamin C per day for six weeks will be beneficial for healing.

Calcium and vitamin D

Calcium is a mineral that is essential to build and maintain strong teeth and bones, and for muscle control and blood circulation. Calcium is not made in the body, but rather absorbed from the foods we eat. In order to absorb calcium from our food, our body needs vitamin D. The amount of calcium needed per day varies between 1,000–1,300 mg based on age. Adolescents, postmenopausal women and men older than 70 require more calcium.

Vitamin D is needed to absorb calcium for good bone health. Recently it has been recommended that our body needs at least 1,000 IU of vitamin D per day for good bone health, beginning at the age of 5.

Building muscle mass via diet

Exercise is important to build muscle mass. But how can you gain more muscle mass with less time for training? The secret is in nutrition.

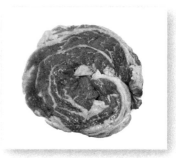

Here is a list of the top 10 foods to build muscle mass.

1. Lean beef
2. Skinless chicken
3. Cottage cheese
4. Fish
5. Whey protein
6. Eggs
7. Oatmeal
8. Fruits and vegetables
9. Whole grains
10. Healthy fats including nuts, flaxseed oil, avocados and seeds

Omega-3 fatty acids

For normal growth and development, omega-3 fatty acids are essential. Since our bodies are unable to make omega-3s, they must come from our diets. Fats are important for reducing inflammation.

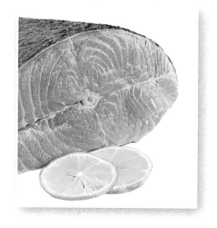

Omega-3s are found in walnuts, soybeans, tofu, flaxseed, canola oil, avocados, olive oil, cod liver, and cold-water fish such as tuna and salmon. The American Heart Association recommends 1 gram per day of eicosapentaenoic acid (EPA) and docosehexaenoic acid (DHA) for patients with heart disease; they also recommend eating fish twice a week for maintenance. In patients with heart disease, it would appear that omega-3 fatty acids reduce cellular aging.

There is strong evidence that omega-3s can lower blood pressure and bad (LDL) cholesterol. There are studies that suggest omega-3 fatty acids benefit patients with autoimmune conditions, such as rheumatoid arthritis. Inadequate supply of omega-3 fatty acids results in bone loss and degeneration of the spine may be delayed by high doses. However, these high doses may result in bleeding. Anyone considering this should consult their physician.

One risk of taking omega-3 fatty acid supplements is gastrointestinal upset. People who are pregnant, diabetic, on blood thinners, on anti-inflammatories (Advil, Aleve, Motrin), or taking ginko biloda should consult a physician.

It is important to remember that not all fats are equal. Trans fats, omega-6 fats and saturated fats may hinder healing by increasing inflammation.

Glucosamine and chondroitin

The cartilage of a joint is the cushion or gliding surface that separates bones to form a joint. Glucosamine and chondroitin are part of normal cartilage. Glucosamine is a natural substance that is found covering shellfish and is easily absorbed by the body. Chondroitin is found in shark or bovine cartilage, and can also be made in a laboratory.

Glucosamine and chondroitin are supplements frequently taken for arthritis. Some people think it helps slow arthritis, but to date there have been no scientific studies that demonstrate the slowing of joint destruction. Some studies have shown that glucosamine eases the pain of mild to moderate osteoarthritis of the knee. A new randomized controlled clinical trial has provided some support for the suggestion raised in the 2008 Glucosamine/Chondroitin Arthritis Intervention Trial (GAIT) that glucosamine and chondroitin sulfate might provide clinically significant pain relief for patients with moderate to severe knee osteoarthritis (OA) pain, despite being ineffective against milder OA pain.

Generally, glucosamine and chondroitin are safe, although people with a shellfish allergy should avoid them. Women who are pregnant or breast-feeding should also avoid them.

If you are considering taking these supplements, discuss it with your physician and remember the supplements are not standardized or regulated by the FDA.

Weight management

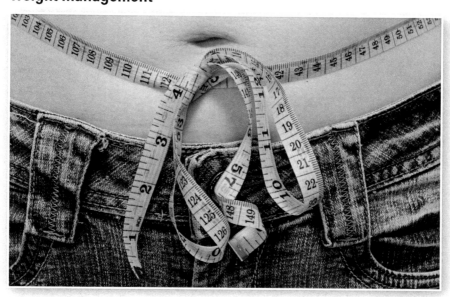

As weight increases, back pain and extremity arthritis increases. There are approximately 125 million adults in America and 65 percent of them are categorized as overweight or obese.

Obesity is defined based on a body mass index (BMI). BMI is closely related to both the percentage of body fat and total body fat. BMI can be found by dividing your mass by the square of your height. Visit www.bmi-calculator.net to calculate your BMI.

Body Mass Index Table

	Normal						Overweight						Obese										Extreme Obesity														
BMI	19	20	21	22	23	24	25	26	27	28	29	30	31	32	33	34	35	36	37	38	39	40	41	42	43	44	45	46	47	48	49	50	51	52	53	54
Height (inches)																	Body Weight (pounds)																			
58	91	96	100	105	110	115	119	124	129	134	138	143	148	153	158	162	167	172	177	181	186	191	196	201	205	210	215	220	224	229	234	239	244	248	253	258
59	94	99	104	109	114	119	124	128	133	138	143	148	153	158	163	168	173	178	183	188	193	198	203	208	212	217	222	227	232	237	242	247	252	257	262	267
60	97	102	107	112	118	123	128	133	138	143	148	153	158	163	168	174	179	184	189	194	199	204	209	215	220	225	230	235	240	245	250	255	261	266	271	276
61	100	106	111	116	122	127	132	137	143	148	153	158	164	169	174	180	185	190	195	201	206	211	217	222	227	232	238	243	248	254	259	264	269	275	280	285
62	104	109	115	120	126	131	136	142	147	153	158	164	169	175	180	186	191	196	202	207	213	218	224	229	235	240	246	251	256	262	267	273	278	284	289	295
63	107	113	118	124	130	135	141	146	152	158	163	169	175	180	186	191	197	203	208	214	220	225	231	237	242	248	254	259	265	270	278	282	287	293	299	304
64	110	116	122	128	134	140	145	151	157	163	169	174	180	186	192	197	204	209	215	221	227	232	238	244	250	256	262	267	273	279	285	291	296	302	308	314
65	114	120	126	132	138	144	150	156	162	168	174	180	186	192	198	204	210	216	222	228	234	240	246	252	258	264	270	276	282	288	294	300	306	312	318	324
66	118	124	130	136	142	148	155	161	167	173	179	186	192	198	204	210	216	223	229	235	241	247	253	260	266	272	278	284	291	297	303	309	315	322	328	334
67	121	127	134	140	146	153	159	166	172	178	185	191	198	204	211	217	223	230	236	242	249	255	261	268	274	280	287	293	299	306	312	319	325	331	338	344
68	125	131	138	144	151	158	164	171	177	184	190	197	203	210	216	223	230	236	243	249	256	262	269	276	282	289	295	302	308	315	322	328	335	341	348	354
69	128	135	142	149	155	162	169	176	182	189	196	203	209	216	223	230	236	243	250	257	263	270	277	284	291	297	304	311	318	324	331	338	345	351	358	365
70	132	139	146	153	160	167	174	181	188	195	202	209	216	222	229	236	243	250	257	264	271	278	285	292	299	306	313	320	327	334	341	348	355	362	369	376
71	136	143	150	157	165	172	179	186	193	200	208	215	222	229	236	243	250	257	265	272	279	286	293	301	308	315	322	329	338	343	351	358	365	372	379	386
72	140	147	154	162	169	177	184	191	199	206	213	221	228	235	242	250	258	265	272	279	287	294	302	309	316	324	331	338	346	353	361	368	375	383	390	397
73	144	151	159	166	174	182	189	197	204	212	219	227	235	242	250	257	265	272	280	288	295	302	310	318	325	333	340	348	355	363	371	378	386	393	401	408
74	148	155	163	171	179	186	194	202	210	218	225	233	241	249	256	264	272	280	287	295	303	311	319	326	334	342	350	358	365	373	381	389	396	404	412	420
75	152	160	168	176	184	192	200	208	216	224	232	240	248	256	264	272	279	287	295	303	311	319	327	335	343	351	359	367	375	383	391	399	407	415	423	431
76	156	164	172	180	189	197	205	213	221	230	238	246	254	263	271	279	287	295	304	312	320	328	336	344	353	361	369	377	385	394	402	410	418	426	435	443

Source: Adapted from Clinical Guidelines on the Identification, Evaluation, and Treatment of Overweight and Obesity in Adults: The Evidence Report.

A BMI of 18.5–24.9 is normal, 25–29.9 is overweight, 30–34.9 is obese, and a BMI greater than 35 is morbidly obese. Compared to those in the normal category, people with a BMI between 25–29 reported 20 percent more pain, those between 30–34 reported 68 percent more pain, 35–39 reported 136 percent more pain, and those with a BMI over 40 reported 254 percent more pain. It is clear to see that, as size increases, pain also increases.

Extra weight will increase pressure on the spine and extremities, and accelerates the wearing out of discs, ligaments and joints. The wearing out of joints results in osteoarthritis.

The main treatment for obesity is dieting and physical exercise. When starting an exercise program, the general rule is to move as much as you can without pain. Try to do it every day and build up to one hour per day. Low impact exercises like walking or using a stationary bike are a good place to start. But if you are weight-bearing intolerant, then a swimming program is the only place to start. If you are unable to progress via traditional means, then the most effective treatment would be bariatric surgery. Bariatric surgery may be either lap band, gastric sleeve, or G.I. bypass surgery, but you should consult a bariatric surgeon for full discussion.

People with obesity are not subjected to increased surgical complications because of their large physical size. However, the obese patient with significant medical comorbidities (diabetes, hypertension, heart disease, sleep apnea, etc.) does have a higher percentage of complications based on the magnitude of their diseases.

Generally, the effects of obesity on low back pain can be reversed, as long as it is addressed prior to doing irreversible damage to your back (eg. spinal stenosis, spondylolisthesis, disc herniations, or radiculopathy). Between 20–30 percent of people who are morbidly obese and have a BMI more than 45 live 13–20 years less than people with a normal BMI. Women of the same age and BMI will shorten their lives by five to eight years. So once you become morbidly obese (or more than 100 pounds over ideal body weight) not only will your life be shortened, you will develop irreversible damage to your spine and other joints, and have more pain. Become committed to life and good health today.

SURGERY

In order for people of different worlds to understand each other, it is important that communication is the common ground. Having a conversation to obtain relevant information forms the basis to answers. This takes patience and time. Sometimes busy people working in their own little space fail to recognize the bigger picture.

Making a decision about health care is one of the most important decisions of your life. Proactive decision-making can give you a greater degree of control over treatment. You should be thoroughly informed about your diagnosis, prognosis, available treatment options, risks/complications and anticipated outcomes.

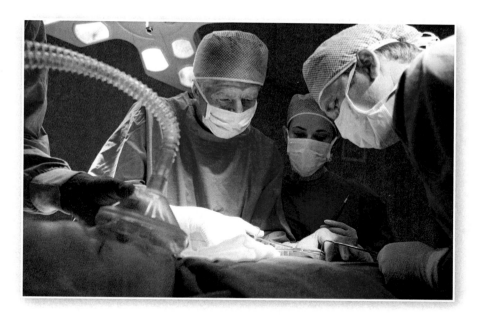

A good doctor will understand your rights to be well informed and should be supportive of a second opinion. Get all of your medical records and diagnostic studies to share with your second doctor. Understand that opinions may differ. Factors that affect opinions include technology, school of thought, where training was obtained, individual methods of treatment, and experience dealing with a particular situation. You must also recognize that there are various treatment methods. Your doctor may choose to treat a pathology one way, while the history of the pathology may be such that a more invasive treatment would result in a better long-term outcome.

Getting a second opinion is never a bad idea. If the first doctor's opinion is the same or similar to the second opinion, then you should be confident in the opinion. Should opinions differ, further investigation may be needed. Studies have shown that 30 percent of patients who sought a second opinion for elective surgery found that the opinions were not in agreement.

Choosing a physician is extremely important. Gather objective information and do not be swayed by the latest and greatest medical craze. **Try to focus on the gold standard of care as this will result in a more predictable outcome.** Also, recognize that some doctors are more conservative while others tend to be more aggressive. Regardless, be aware of long-term outcome data pertaining to the treatment option. After all that is what you want — your surgery to last.

Minimally invasive surgery

Minimally invasive orthopedic surgery was introduced via arthroscopy, which was developed by professor Kenji Takagi in 1919. In arthroscopy a small scope is introduced into a joint for diagnosis or therapeutic reasons. In 1939, Gerhard Kuntscher introduced the use of an intramedullary nail for long bone fractures by a smaller incision, which helped further develop minimally invasive surgery techniques.

Performing minimally invasive spine surgery is like building a ship in a bottle. The term minimally invasive describes surgical procedures that are performed through small incisions or openings to gain access to a 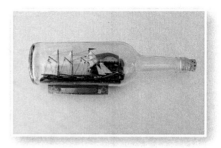 specific part of the body. The purpose of minimally invasive surgery is to reduce damage to surrounding tissues, speed up healing and recover with less pain.

Advantages:

- ➤ Quicker return to activities
- ➤ Smaller incision
- ➤ Less damage to surrounding muscle
- ➤ Potentials for less blood loss, shorter hospital stay, quicker healing and potentially less pain

Disadvantages:

- ➤ Steep learning curve
- ➤ Potential for prolonged operative times
- ➤ Increased radiation exposure
- ➤ Not appropriate for every case
- ➤ Difficult to apply bone for fusion cases
- ➤ Difficult to repair a spinal fluid leak

Minimally invasive techniques for spine surgery have been used since the 1990s predominantly for decompressions and limited fusions. Newer techniques are currently being developed to push the envelope and perform internal fixation, but remember that it is still spine surgery.

CASE STUDY:
Samuel L. Jackson

An actor known for a wide-range of roles, Samuel Jackson's movies include *Shaft*, *Pulp Fiction*, and the *Star Wars* prequels. While filming *S.W.A.T.*, Jackson says he woke up one morning and could not move. He rolled out of bed, crawled to the bathroom, took some Advil, and eventually ended up getting an epidural steroid injection so he could finish the movie. When it wrapped, he had to have a cyst removed from his sciatic nerve.

To achieve a pain-free status, he reports undergoing regular acupuncture sessions (twice per week) and having a titanium bolt put in his spine, which was fitted to allow him to walk, bend over and even play golf.

In 2012, the FDA approved the Coflex ® Interlaminar Stabilization ™ device (Paradigm Spine, New York). The device offers motion preserving, non-fusion stabilization after a surgical decompression for moderate-to-sever spinal stenosis. Jackson appeared on *The Ellen Show* in 2015 to relate his experience with the device and how it has helped relieve his back issues.

The use of minimally invasive orthopedic surgery has been introduced over the past 100 years as technology has been developed. Now the conversion from inpatient to 24-hour stay to outpatient surgery is occurring as new technologies, techniques and medications are becoming available.

Outpatient, or ambulatory, surgery is very common in orthopedic surgery. Historically it has occurred in hand, foot and sports medicine surgeries. Now with the introduction of newer medications, surgical techniques and accelerated recovery programs, this innovation has allowed a movement to outpatient surgery for joint replacement and spinal surgery. Spinal surgical procedures that are conducive to outpatient procedures include the smaller cases such as laminectomies, disectomies, foraminotomies, one level anterior cervical fusions, one level transforaminal lumbar interbody fusions, and one level decompression/stabilization procedures.

In order to be a candidate you must be:

> Physiologically younger
> Healthy
> More active
> Motivated
> Able to play hurt

There is currently a greater emphasis on performing less invasive surgeries while trying to mobilize the patient as rapidly as possible. Patient selection is important. Those patients who require more extensive procedures, have medical comorbidities, or require careful postoperative monitoring, will continue to need traditional inpatient hospital settings.

In order to decrease cost, expense, lost time from work, and have a safe procedure, it is important to educate yourself about ambulatory surgery and plan carefully.

Laser surgery

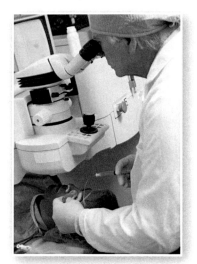

A laser is a device that emits focused light through a process of optical amplification based on the stimulated emission of electromagnetic radiation. In medicine lasers have been used for bloodless surgery, laser healing, dentistry, kidney stone treatment and eye treatment. A laser beam can either cut tissue or vaporize it. The most commonly accepted uses for lasers are in eye surgery, vascular surgery and gastrointestinal tract surgery. There are differences between the use of the laser or scalpel and its use. The three differences are angles of cutting, heat and gas generation, and depth of penetration. In a comparison of the two, the scalpel wins in all categories.

In a recent study by Brouwer et al. comparing percutaneous laser decompression versus conventional micro discectomy in sciatica, laser proved just as effective as traditional surgery. It would thus appear that this surgical procedure could serve as an intermediate intervention between conservative care and surgery.

Although laser spine surgery has gained popularity with the public, at this time many spine experts have not endorsed the technique. Although lasers are FDA approved, laser spine surgery is a technique that is not accepted by most insurance carriers.

Robotic Surgery

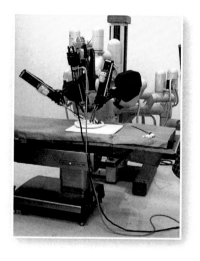

Robotic surgery may be performed using smaller incisions. It was originally designed for general surgery, gynecology and urology. In these procedures the actual operating surgeon is in another room while the robot performs the surgical procedure. Also currently available are navigational devices that are used to provide assistance in the implantation of instrumentation while leaving the actual surgery in the surgeon's hands. Spine surgery is a delicate and potentially hazardous procedure. Oftentimes the procedures are performed on or around the spinal cord, peripheral nerves, or blood vessels. The deviation of millimeters may mean the difference between success and failure.

The development of robotic devices to support all spinal procedures has significant applications. It creates accurate tools, reduced radiation exposure and fewer complications.

The system consists of the following:

➤ Workstation
➤ Planning software
➤ A highly accurate guidance unit (RBT device) that moves in all planes
➤ Several spinal mounting platforms

All this advance technology allows the surgeon to more accurately place instrumentation (which translates into increased safety), make smaller incisions (which means less muscle injury and less blood loss), and ultimately leads to a shorter hospital stay and faster return to home, family and work. While these are still works in progress, they have the potential to make spine surgery safer and less invasive.

HYGIENE AND SHOWERING

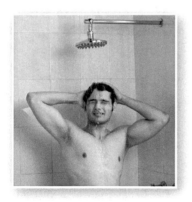

Most dermatologists agree that the average person showers or bathes entirely too much. Most people feel that showering and bathing is mostly for social and aesthetic reasons rather than for health. The concern about oils on the skin and hair growth surpasses concept of prevention of bacterial transmission for the injured.

Around all health care facilities these days you see hand sanitizing dispensers for health care workers to dispense antibacterial solutions to prevent transmission of infection to the ill. From a health care perspective in treating patients with injury or illness, I feel it is of utmost importance to have a daily bath or shower to prevent the transmission of infection, despite what the dermatologists say.

A shower or bath will:

- Reduce muscle tension
- Improve blood circulation
- Boost the immune system
- Lower blood sugars
- Reduce stress
- Improve lung function
- Improve sleep

By using an antibacterial soap with your shower you can decrease the colony count of bacteria on your skin and therefore decrease the potential for an infection. Now postoperative patients have plastic dressings that are not changed for three to five days and allow them to shower. During this period of time the incision will undergo the epithelialization process and the wound will begin to heal. These dressings prevent contamination of the wound, prevent heat loss, maintain an optimal environment for healing and serve as a barrier to external bacterial contamination or cross contamination to others.

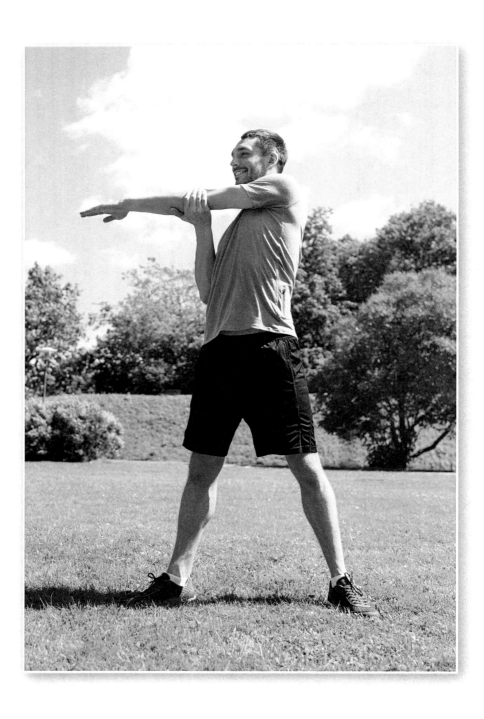

CHAPTER 7

Exercise Programs

RANGE OF MOTION AND STRETCHING

Regaining range of motion of a joint is an important component of injury recovery. Range of motion may be either active or passive. In an active range of motion, or active stretch, you ask the joint to move, and move it according to its ability. In passive range of motion, or passive stretch, you assist the joint in its motion.

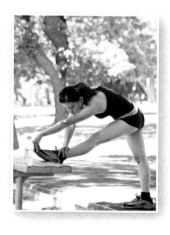

Stretching is an important component of wellness and injury recovery of the musculoskeletal system. Stretching may help improve joint and soft tissue range of motion, which in return will improve performance and decrease risk of injury. Remember the Tin Man in *The Wizard of Oz*? The Tin Man became frozen solid if he did not have lubrication for his joints. In order for your body to create joint fluid the joints need to be mobile. After injury or due to lack of use, joints become stiff. Stretching helps improve flexibility or motion of a joint. Better flexibility will improve performance and decrease risk of reinjury. Stretching also increases blood flow to muscles.

Before stretching, it is important to learn how to stretch properly. Improper stretching may actually be more harmful than not stretching at all. It is important to warm up cold muscles prior to stretching. Any low-level activity, such as walking for five to 10 minutes just to get the blood flow going, is good. When stretching it is important to focus on the muscle groups you wish to stretch as well as the type of joint you are trying to stretch. A knee joint is a hinge joint so it only can go in two directions, whereas a shoulder joint may go in six directions. When stretching, it is important that your movement be smooth without any bouncing. Bouncing may result in further injury to your muscle. Hold each stretch for approximately 30 seconds and try to breathe normally. You should feel a gradual tension but not pain. If pain develops you have overstretched. Stretching may be activity specific; with running sports hamstrings are often the focus. Lastly it is also important to stretch on a regular basis and to incorporate movement into your stretch. The co-ordination of movement with stretch, such as in yoga or tai chi, teaches your muscles how to work in a coordinated fashion.

A joint that is not used can become shortened and stiff. This is most commonly seen in sprains, strains, tendinitis and any overuse syndrome. Restarting joint motion can accelerate recovery from injury by improving circulation, enhancing neurologic injury and increasing nutrient supply to muscle.

Stretching becomes important in an injury recovery program. In the first 72 hours after injury it is important to follow the RICE treatment protocol. Avoid any stretching during the first 72 hours. After 72 hours, start with some general active treatments. These should include the use of heat, massage, and some slow general static and passive stretching exercises. A static stretching exercise is performed by placing the body part being stretched into position and then beginning to stretch under tension. This can be performed slowly and cautiously until a tension is created in the stretched muscle group so as to allow the muscle to lengthen. A passive stretch occurs when another person or apparatus is employed to further the stretch of the muscle. This passive stretch results in a greater force being applied to the muscle and may also be more hazardous. The most important thing to remember is that light gentle stretch is the key. Over the next two to five weeks it is important to regain flexibility, strength, power, balance, muscular endurance and coordination. So in addition to active and passive stretching, you should incorporate proprioceptive neuromuscular facilitation, which involves both stretching and contracting the muscle group targeted.

In the long term, dynamic and active stretching may be incorporated to make an injured area stronger and more flexible than it was before the injury occurred. Dynamic stretching employs a controlled, swinging motion to a specific body part for the full extent of its range of motion. Active stretching involves only using the strength of one's opposing muscles to generate a stretch. Thus the goal of stretching is to allow your body to become loose, limber and pain-free.

STARTING A MOBILIZATION PROGRAM

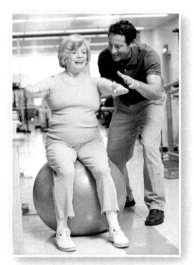

The initiation of an exercise program after injury is important to speed up recovery. Anabolic hormones such as testosterone, growth hormone and IGF-1 are required to make proteins such as muscles, tendons and all other body tissues. So in order to repair the damage after an injury anabolic hormones are required. **The body normally makes these hormones, but as we age they dramatically decrease starting around the age of 25 and then a steep plunge occurs around the age of 40.** Does this remind you of Tiger Woods' scenario? This is why as we age we tend to heal very slowly. So, after the age of 25 if you are injured your options are to accept slow, imperfect healing as a consequence of aging, increase your hormone levels illegally or try to boost your own internal levels of anabolic hormones. The most effective way to boost anabolic hormones is by exercise, in addition to rest and increased protein intake. It has been found that multiple short bursts of exercise throughout the day are more effective in generating anabolic hormones than a single workout. Generally, this can be started with a walking program that increases pace periodically. If your injury is to your arm, then lifting weights will help. Even if you are confined to a hospital bed, simply lifting some books is a good start. The bottom line is that whatever you can do without reinjuring yourself will result in your body's manufacturing of anabolic hormones, which will aid in allowing you to heal faster and more completely.

WALKING PROGRAM

Trying to start or maintain a physical activity program? Trying to lose weight? Ever think about getting some objective data? Recently, physical activity monitors have been introduced. The monitor is a small flexible band that fits on your wrist. It syncs with your computer and works like a pedometer, but better. The objective is to take 10,000 steps per day, which translates into approximately 4 miles. When the person reaches 10,000 steps the device vibrates. By syncing it with your cellphone/computer you can monitor your progress every week.

Remember that this is only a device that tracks activity level. It is a start. It can also be a motivational tool to do better than you did the day before. Try it. You may like it, and it may motivate you. There are also advanced devices that monitor not only the number of steps you have taken, but also the number of flights of steps, your heart rate, hours of sleep and calories taken in/burned.

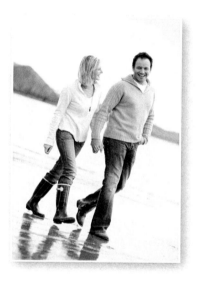

THERAPEUTIC EXERCISE

The incorporation of therapeutic exercise into a rehabilitation program is extremely important unless your physician directs otherwise. Therapeutic exercise helps to reduce pain and increases function in nearly all musculoskeletal injuries. But not all rehabilitation programs are the same. Occasionally a program is not successful. If that appears to be the way you are heading, here are some suggestions to prevent failure.

Here are some considerations to explain program failure:

> Inaccurate initial assessment
> Lack of secondary assessments
> Poor exercise techniques
> Lack of multidisciplinary approach
> Poor supervision
> Lack of modification of exercise for progression
> Outdated techniques
> Poor engagement

MOVE IT PROGRAM

The move it program is designed to be proactive, so you can feel better and be healthy.

Arthritis affects cartilage, which is the smooth protective tissue that covers bones where they meet and allows them to glide and move easily. When you develop arthritis, the cartilage wears away, the bone rubs together, and it makes it hard to move. When joints do not move, the tendons and muscles around the joint stiffen and become painful when the joint is moved.

You can learn to manage arthritis and protect your joints through a three part plan, which involes getting stronger to move better, dropping a few pounds and protecting your joints.

In order to get stronger and move better, you must focus on four types of exercise; muscle strengthening, aerobics, core and flexibility. The best results from your time and effort can be obtained by taking small steps when starting, gradually doing more a little bit at a time, and always warming up and cooling down for any kind of exercise.

Strengthening exercises should be done three days/week in 15–30 minute sessions. Flexibility stretches should be done seven days/week for five minutes/day. Aerobics/cardio activity should be three days/week for five to 30 minutes progressing to a daily routine as you get healthier. Aerobic exercise (walking, dancing, exercise class) is usually weight-bearing exercise. Non-weight-bearing exercises (swimming, water aerobics, and bike riding) are for those patients who are weight-bearing intolerant so they can get started and gradually work up to weight-bearing exercise.

Swimming

Swimming is an exercise that you may enjoy throughout your entire life. It is a low impact activity that has many physical and mental health benefits. Additionally it is a great workout as you are able to move your whole body against the resistance of water.

The benefits of swimming include:

- ➤ It is a cardio exercise
- ➤ It is a non-weight-bearing
- ➤ Improves endurance, muscle strength and cardiovascular fitness
- ➤ Tones muscles and build strength
- ➤ Total body workout
- ➤ Has a cooling effect
- ➤ Improves flexibility
- ➤ Improves endurance
- ➤ Increases circulation
- ➤ Rehabilitates injured muscles
- ➤ Helps control weight

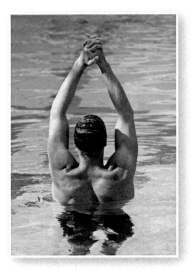

Exercise options include the following:

- ➤ Water walking
- ➤ Water aerobics
- ➤ Water toning/strength toning
- ➤ Flexibility
- ➤ Training water therapy
- ➤ Water yoga and relaxation
- ➤ Deep water running
- ➤ Wall exercises
- ➤ Water fitness products
- ➤ Swimming laps

Swimming gives your body a total workout without all of the harsh impacts. Try it by yourself or in a class.

Balance exercises

Balance exercises are important. Working on a balancing act can activate deep core muscles to help tighten the midsection. It also prepares athletes for a quick turn or lunge. What is good for the athlete is also good for the senior.

People over the age of 65 are more prone to falls, which can result in hip or spine fracture. If a senior falls, it could limit his or her activities and make it impossible to live independently. Balancing exercises along with certain strength exercises can prevent falls.

Basic balance exercises include standing on one foot, walking heel to toe, back and side leg raises, and balance walking. Advanced balance training includes using a BOSU balance trainer, TheraBand, balance board, wobble board, agility ladder, foam roller and slide board.

Some of the benefits of balance training are:

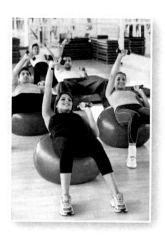

> An increased integration of the nervous system
> Injury prevention
> Injury rehabilitation
> Increased hand-eye coordination
> Improved balance
> Increased muscle activation and recruitment
> Improved performance

A Swiss ball, physio ball or exercise ball is an exercise treatment option for back pain sufferers. This exercise program, designed around the Swiss ball, is used to prevent or minimize further episodes of low back pain and help stabilize the spine. These exercises were designed to introduce an element of instability and exercise muscles that would not be exercised in floor activity. The development of balance and body awareness using the Swiss ball makes muscles even stronger.

Fitness for seniors

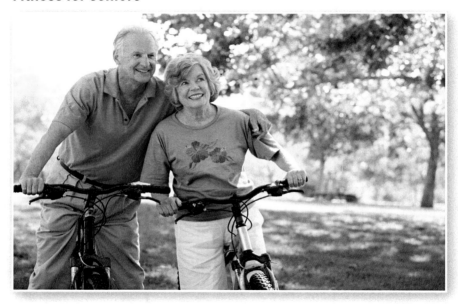

Keeping active and remaining fit can help prolong your life and even prevent or delay illnesses or disabilities as you grow older. The benefits of physical activity extend throughout life and can improve many health conditions. Being active helps lower your risk of falls and developing heart disease and diabetes. It can even help you live on your own longer. Fitness and physical activity are safe for seniors — even those with stable chronic conditions, such as heart disease, diabetes and arthritis. Your doctor can offer advice about the safety of certain activities and increasing your fitness level. The Journal of the American Medical Association published an article about how daily activity levels in healthy older adults aged 70 to 82 years are associated with longevity.

How to keep fit:

➤ Choose activities you enjoy.
➤ Make being fit part of your everyday life. Playing with children, gardening, walking, dancing and housekeeping are just a few activities that can improve your fitness.
➤ Combine a range of activities that include aerobics, strengthening exercises, flexibility and balance.
➤ Start slow and gradually build up to a total of at least 30 minutes of activity a day on most days of the week. Activities can be broken up throughout the day.
➤ Keep safety in mind. Always wear comfortable, well-fitting shoes and use appropriate safety gear. Avoid outdoor activities in extreme cold or heat.
➤ Drink plenty of fluids while engaging in physical activity.

Types of activities seniors can perform are aerobic activities, strengthening activities, flexibility and balancing activities. Aerobic exercises are those that increase oxygen use to improve heart and lung function and include activities such as walking, gardening, and swimming. They can help strengthen your heart, lower your blood pressure and cholesterol, and improve your mood and sleep. Strengthening activities (such as repetitive lifting of light weights or even household items such as canned foods) can improve your muscle and bone health. Strengthening leg and hip muscles with leg weight exercises can help reduce your risk of falls. Flexibility and balancing activities (such as tai chi, stretching and yoga) can help prevent injuries and stiff joints.

Stop the activity and call your doctor if you experience any of the following symptoms:

- ➤ Pain or pressure in your chest, arms, neck, or jaw
- ➤ Feeling light headed, nauseated, or weak
- ➤ Becoming short of breath
- ➤ Developing pain in your legs, calves, or back
- ➤ Having an uncomfortable sensation of your heart beating too fast

For a senior, any physical activity is better than none. The U.S. guidelines for people over age 60 show moderate to vigorous exercise was linked to a 28 percent decrease risk of dying over a 10-year period compared to those who were completely sedentary. Even low levels of exercise were linked to a 22 percent decrease in death. It is thus recommended that seniors attempt to perform 150 minutes per week of moderate to vigorous exercise. Exercise is calculated by metabolic equivalent of tasks or METs. METs represent the amount of energy expended per minute in a specific activity. For example, resting results in one MET, moderate activities, such as walking, use three to six METs, and vigorous exercise such as running uses more than six METs. A weekly exercise regime is low if it totaled one to 499 METs, moderate at 500–999 METs, and high if it reached more than 1,000 METs.

The mortality rate is 22 percent lower for people with low METs, 28 percent lower for people with moderate to vigorous exercise, and for those who expended at least 1,000 METs per week there was a 35 percent lower mortality rate. Therefore researchers recommend 15 minutes per day of exercise in order to decrease the mortality risk from cardiovascular disease.

CASE STUDY:
Klaus Obermeyer

In 1947, Klaus Obermeyer arrived in Aspen, Colorado where he spent the next 12 years working as a ski instructor. He founded Sport Obermeyer and led innovations such as a down ski parka stitched together from a down comforter. As a ski enthusiast and entrepreneur, he has spent his life contributing to the sport of skiing, and at age 96, he has reported no thoughts of retiring.

Even though age does eventually take its toll on the body, maintaining a fit, active lifestyle can stem off many of the signs of aging. Obermeyer reports that he still skis every winter day that the weather is good and leads the way in taking advantage of a company policy that states if there is six inches of snow or more, staff can hit the slopes in the morning and come to work later in the day.

Yet, Obermeyer does not just get his activity on the slopes; he has also pursued the Japanese martial art, aikido, for the last 35 years. He contributes this as well as his time swimming to his vitality and physical well-being. Not surprisingly, Obermeyer also maintains a strict diet that includes a hearty breakfast, fresh fruit throughout the day, and a light dinner rich in greens. "I try to be vegan, but I'm a vegan who cheats," he said. "My main concern is not to eat more calories than I burn."

Fit moms

After having a baby a woman's body changes. But getting your body back is not as hard
as you might think. Regular exercise is good
for your general health, but after giving birth
exercise becomes essential to reduce the risk
of postpartum depression.

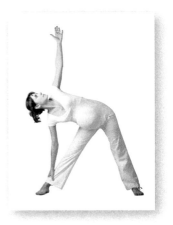

Here are some tips to begin your exercise
program and recover your body:

> ➤ Start a walking program
> ➤ Begin deep belly breathing with abdominal contractures
> ➤ Practice head lifts, shoulder lifts and curl ups
> ➤ Try kneeling pelvic tilts
> ➤ Do forward and side lunges
> ➤ Do squats

Try to do as many exercises as possible with your baby in a baby carrier
or wrap. This adds weight to your workout, works on balance and allows for the bonding that mothers and babies need. Do these workouts
in a class for an additional benefit.

Core stability

It used to be believed that the core of an apple had seeds that contain amygdalin. This substance can release cyanide when in contact with digestive enzymes. Therefore it was believed that eating the core of an apple could be lethal. Scientists have since determined that this is indeed a myth. It is safe to eat an occasional apple core. Just as the apple core has had a history of being poorly understood, likewise core stability is misunderstood.

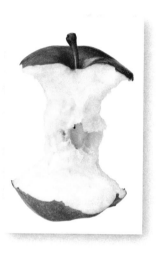

The core refers to the body region bounded by the abdominal wall, the pelvis, the lower back and the diaphragm. The core has the unique ability to stabilize the body during movement. The core consists of the abdominal muscle groups, hip abductors, hip flexors, the pelvic floor and lumbar spine. This combination is responsible for posture, stability and strength, which are all especially needed for dynamic sports.

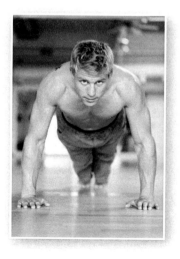

Training methods for developing and maintaining core stability include Pilates and using a Swiss exercise ball. A simple exercise used to strengthen the abdominals is the well-known plank. The plank stimulates the need to resist movement and focuses on spinal stability. An exercise called contralateral bird-dog, where you keep a neutral spine and increase intra-abdominal pressure before performing movement, is also used to strengthen the abdominals. In general, these core specific exercises seem to have the same benefits as general, nonspecific exercises and walking. The core stability model consists of both passive and active stabilization and training of the neuromotor system. This training should provide rather quick responses to the body's demands. Athletes who need to cut quickly should employ these techniques.

It is believed that inefficient core stability can result in lower back pain, poor posture and lethargy. Yet there is little support in research for the core stability model and its ability to prevent injury and improve performance.

Core strengthening is a good concept, but the idea of preventing spinal injury through core strengthening is cloaked in myth just like the core of the apple.

Lifting weights

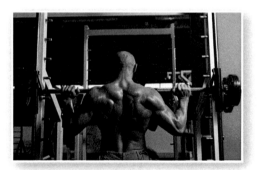

There are four types of exercise — cardio, core strengthening, flexibility and weight training. Weight training is a common type of strength training in which the goal is to increase the strength and size of skeletal muscle. This type of exercise usually involves the lifting of weights. By using a weight against the force of gravity, you stimulate a concentric or eccentric contraction of the muscle to strengthen that muscle. These exercises are designed to increase physical strength.

In order to get maximum benefits you should:

> ➤ Employ proper technique
> ➤ Properly warm-up
> ➤ Breathe properly
> ➤ Stay hydrated
> ➤ Carefully plan sets and reps
> ➤ Avoid injury by avoiding pain

Free weights versus weight machines

Free weights are non-constraining. They may be used in various positions and require the use of stabilizer muscles. Weight machines, on the other hand, are more restrictive, but they enforce better form and may help prevent injury.

It would appear that free weights have more benefits for the experienced weightlifter, whereas the recreational weightlifter is safer with the weight machines. The overall benefits of weight training include increased muscle mass, strength, endurance, bone formation and a whole host of metabolic benefits for overall health.

Elliptical trainer

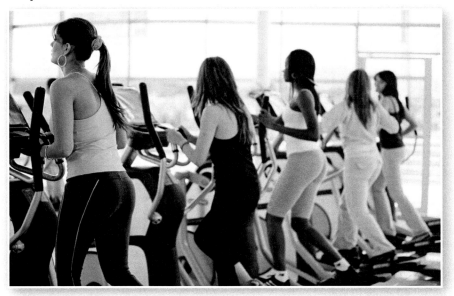

An elliptical trainer is a stationary exercise machine that simulates walking, running or stair climbing without causing excessive stress on the body's joints. By decreasing stress, the goal is to decrease the potential for exercise-induced injury. Elliptical trainers offer a cardiovascular workout that is low impact. You can vary the intensity, speed of exercise and resistance to accommodate individual goals.

Elliptical trainers were invented by Precor in the 1990s. Studies have shown that as stride is lengthened, more calories are burned and a larger variety of muscle groups are employed. This low-impact type of exercise is very user friendly.

Running

Running is an exercise that involves repetitive stress and impact. Whether it is a short jog or a longer run, it is generally found that running or jogging makes low back problems worse. Additionally, if injury to the spine occurs, sciatica (leg pain, weakness, or numbness) may result.

Studies by Garbutt and colleagues measured the stress on the back while running. They found a significant correlation between spinal shrinkage, running speed and distance covered to the effect that the longer and faster you run the shorter you get (temporarily). After a 30 minute run it was found that the height of a runner dropped by more than a quarter of an inch. This decrease in height had no correlation with a history of back pain. It appears that for the recreational athlete that the spine is well-equipped to handle the loads incurred with running.

Other studies have been performed on elite athletes that found low back pain was significantly less common in these athletes than in the general population. Alternatively, according to MRI studies, weightlifters and soccer players have an increased rate of disc degeneration, which was not the case with long-time runners.

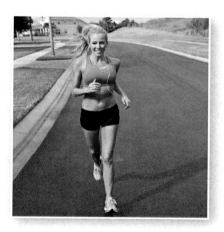

It appears that runners have healthier backs than sedentary people and weightlifting athletes.

Yoga

Yoga is an ancient practice developed in India almost 4,000 years ago. In the last decade yoga has significantly increased in popularity, with about 15 million people in the United States performing yoga. U.S. yoga classes are a combination of breathing exercises, physical exercise and meditation.

The primary benefits of yoga are:

➤ Learning relaxation and acceptance
➤ Relieving pain
➤ Increasing strength and flexibility

Hatha yoga is one branch of yoga and consists of physical postures (asanas), breathing techniques (pranayama) and meditation. Several studies have demonstrated that it is effective for reducing pain and improving function. Iyengar yoga is a form of Hatha yoga that focuses on detail, precision and alignment in the performance of posture and breathing control. Strength, mobility and stability are developed through posture. Iyengar yoga is considered to be therapeutic, quasi-medical yoga and effective for many treatments of medical conditions. The general concept regarding a sequence of yoga poses is predetermined by a strict order, with appropriate preparation devoted for inversions and back extensions. Sequencing, timing and intricacy of the poses provide a framework to structure the progression and content of the therapy.

Adho Mukha Svanasana
(Downward-facing dog pose)

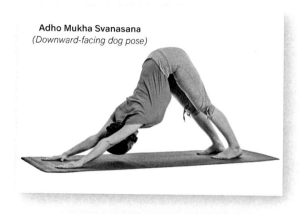

Utthita Trikonasana
(Extended triangle pose)

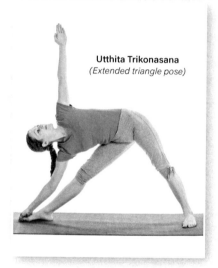

Prasarita Padottanasana
(Intense leg stretch)

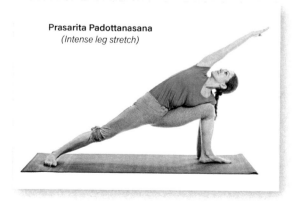

Physical benefits of yoga exercises:

- ➤ Increased strength from holding yoga positions
- ➤ Allows stretching and relaxation
- ➤ Better posture, balance and body alignment
- ➤ Increased body awareness

Mental benefits of yoga exercises:

- ➤ Reduces stress
- ➤ Enhances mood

One of the primary causes of neck and back pain is muscle tension. As you work through your yoga poses, your muscles will stretch and loosen. Yoga stretches may be enough to help people with neck or back pain related to stress or poor posture. Patients with osteoarthritis and disc herniation can develop adverse effects from yoga, but studies have shown that these may have been independent of yoga.

Below is a list of common specific asanas designed to reduce neck and back pain:

- ➤ Tadasana – Mountain pose with various arm/shoulder positions
- ➤ Ardha Uttanasana – Half forward bend to wall or ledge
- ➤ Chair Bharadvajasana – Seated chair twist
- ➤ Adho Mukho Virasana – Downward-facing hero pose
- ➤ Adho Mukha Svanasana – Downward-facing dog pose
- ➤ Utthita Trikonasana – Extended triangle pose
- ➤ Virabhadasana II – Warrior pose II
- ➤ Utthita Parsvakonasana – Extended side angle pose
- ➤ Prasarita Padottanasana – Intense leg stretch

- Supta Padangustasana – Reclining big toe (and variations)
- Prone Savasana – Lying prone corpse pose (with weights)
- Supta Pavanamuktasana – Lying both knees to chest pose
- Supta Savasana – Lying supine corpse pose

It is advisable that anyone with a medical condition discuss their situation with the teacher prior to the class. Yoga teacher training and certification are not strictly regulated so it is important to find a yoga teacher experienced with spine problems

Tai chi

Tai chi is an internal Chinese martial art practiced both for defense training and health benefits. It has both hard and soft martial art techniques, demonstration competitions and longevity. Both traditional and modern forms exist.

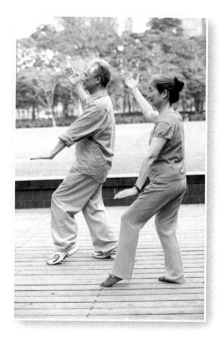

The purpose of tai chi is to focus the mind solely on the movements of the form, which help to bring about a state of mental calm and clarity. This results in both general health benefits and stress management.

The study of tai chi primarily involves three aspects:

1. Health
2. Meditation
3. Martial arts

Training techniques involve:

➤ Solo form
➤ Partnered form
➤ Weapons

Tai chi has been found to help prevent falls and benefit mental and general health in the elderly.

Gyrotonic

Gyrotonic is a type of exercise that involves the use of special equipment, including weights and pulleys. It combines the principles of swimming, yoga, tai chi and dance. Gyrotonic is said to encourage the development of strong muscles, improved flexibility and coordination.

The Gyrotonic Expansion System was created by Juliu Horvath a Romanian raised Hungarian ballet dancer who was also competitive in swimming and gymnastics. He moved to the United States in the 1960s and continued a career in ballet. After a career ending injury, he developed a series of movements and physical activities that mimic dance, gymnastics and swimming. He felt it was important that these movements be low-impact, so as to allow for injury recovery. The exercises are performed on a Gyrotonic machine, which has a tower, a bench, pulleys and straps. These exercises teach elongation and help people regain elasticity in the spine. They focus on arching, curling and twisting motions, which are not routinely performed in everyday life anymore.

Personal training

When should you work with a personal trainer? And when should you work with a personal trainer when you have or have had an injury?

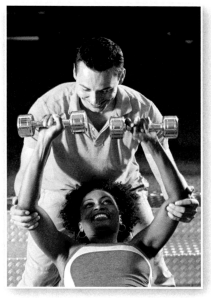

With a personal trainer you can develop new interests and learn to modify your workout to accommodate your injury. Finding a good trainer is most important; a bad trainer can worsen your condition. A good trainer is someone who is knowledgeable, able to effectively communicate, available to answer questions and likeable. As you can see, when creating an exercise program it is important that your trainer has the right skills —just like your doctor.

Remember that a personal fitness trainer designs exercise programs for their clients, while a physical therapist diagnoses, treats and manages pain, injuries and illness with a doctor's order. A physical therapist also has a state license to practice.

Gym and spine pain

Eighty percent of Americans experience spine pain at some point in their lives. At any given time, 31 million Americans are dealing with lower back pain. Most doctors recommend physical activity as a component of treatment for neck and back pain. When you looks out over the gym and see a lot of equipment, it is easy to become intimidated. The question is, what is good for you and what can make you worse?

If you are not in pain and just want to condition there are four components of exercise:

1. Cardio
2. Muscle strengthening
3. Stretching
4. Core strengthening

If you have debilitating pain such that any activity makes symptoms worse, try one of the following:

1. Aqua jogging
2. Swimming
3. Water aerobics

If you are pain-free in a seated position, try one of the following:

1. Controlled motion of weight machines
2. Body weight exercises
3. Recumbent bicycle

Exercises to avoid when you have spine pain:

1. Repetitive bending at the waist
2. Holding a free weight away from your body
3. Holding a weight above your trunk
4. Any exercise that is painful
5. Precor or CrossFit

With a smart training plan, there is no reason for you to gain weight or become deconditioned after an injury.

CrossFit

CrossFit is a company based on a philosophy of physical exercise and competitive fitness. It was started in 2000 by Greg Glassman and Lauren Jenai. CrossFit workouts consist of aerobic exercise, Olympic weight lifting and gymnastics. What is different about this program as opposed to a traditional gym class is that the workout is constantly varied among functional movements performed at a high intensity.

Studies have demonstrated that CrossFit increases cardiovascular and respiratory endurance, strength, power, speed, balance and coordination. Critics have shown that with improper technique, spinal injuries and rhabdomyolysis, the rapid deterioration of muscle tissue, may occur.

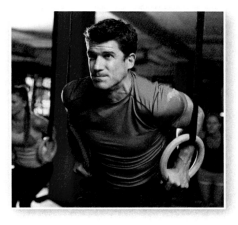

Exercise in the heat

Sweating is good for your body. It keeps you safe during your workout and improves performance. When your body heats up, it converts a chemical energy to work energy and the byproduct is sweat. Sweat keeps body temperature evenly regulated between 98 and 103 F. If body temperature elevates beyond 103 F, performance will suffer and eventually you risk heat exhaustion or worse.

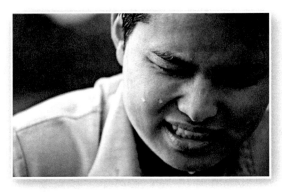

After copious sweating it is important to replace water and other nutrients. It is recommended to consume 20 ounces of liquid for every 45–60 minutes of moderate to intense exercise. After 90 minutes of exercise some sugar and electrolytes are needed. Training in overly heated areas is one way to increase your blood plasma volume, but it comes at a price: increased fluid consumption. A general rule is to replace liquids at a rate of one pint of fluids for every pound lost.

Everyone sweats during exercise. The amount of sweat differs from person to person. Women generally have more sweat glands but sweat less due to less muscle mass. Athletes tend to sweat sooner and more. Overweight or obese people tend to sweat more because of thicker layers of fat that insulate the body.

Exercising in hot weather can be fun but also dangerous. Exercising in the heat puts an added stress on your body. If you are not careful, you can run the risk of coming down with a heat-related illness.

The body has a self-regulating mechanism that attempts to cool your body when you are overheated. The body sends more blood from your muscles to your skin. This alternate flow of blood results in an increased heart rate and an elevated body temperature. Under normal conditions, perspiration will adjust for body temperature. If you do not drink enough fluid or are unable to control your body temperature, then heat-related illness occurs.

Heat-related illnesses include:

> Heat cramps
> Fainting
> Heat exhaustion
> Heatstroke

Signs and symptoms include:

> Confusion
> Irritability
> Heart rhythm problems
> Nausea
> Dizziness
> Fatigue
> Changes in vision
> Muscle cramps

Should you develop any of the above symptoms stop exercising immediately and get out of the heat. Remove extra clothing, and try to cool your body down by drinking cool fluids. If your symptoms do not improve within 30 minutes, seek medical attention immediately.

8

New Shoes and Inserts for Recovery

The cause of musculoskeletal pain most often is multifactorial. Causes may range from degeneration or aging to improper shoes. If you are experiencing musculoskeletal pain while you are standing, walking or running then consider your shoes or the gait pattern you produce. If you are wearing the wrong shoe, the chain of reaction will transfer all the way from your feet to your spine.

Approximately 50 percent of working Americans suffer from back pain. Back pain ranks as the No. 2 reason people see a doctor. Sometimes your feet and improper footwear may be the cause of extremity or back pain.

If the foot is biomechanically incompetent, the change of alignment of structures will result in extremity or back pain. The wearing of a shoe that does not give proper support will only make the problem worse. Since the body is erect and all of our weight is placed on the feet, if the feet are poorly aligned this will transmit abnormal forces to the spine. People have different foot types, with the arch taking one of three shapes: pronation, neutral or supination.

Testing your posture:

1. Pick up the shoe you most commonly wear when you are walking
2. Check your shoe to see where the tread is most worn
   a. If the tread is worn mostly on the outside, this is called supination
   b. If the tread is worn mostly on the inside, this is called pronation
   c. If the tread is evenly worn then you have a balanced stride

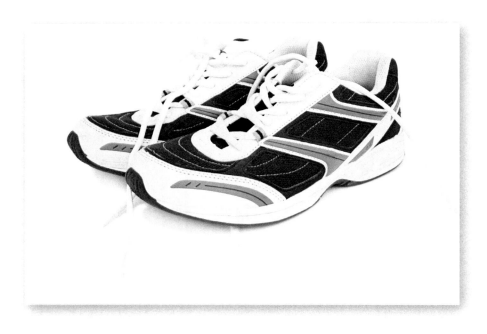

Patients can obtain comfort by the use of running shoes, minimal shoes, inserts or prescription orthotics. Accommodative orthotics are softer and used for support or the cushioning of a painful foot rather than back pain. Functional orthotics are made from either plastic or graphite and are used to treat conditions caused by abnormal motion in the foot. The goal of the insert is for the patient to achieve a healthy posture and gait. As a spine surgeon, I have personally found that accommodative orthotics such as Spenco insoles (Spenco Medical Corp., Waco, Texas), which are relatively inexpensive, provide significant relief for the extremity or back pain patient.

When shopping for new shoes, it is best to shop at the end of the day where your feet are the largest. Measure your feet and try on multiple pairs. There should be half an inch of space from your toe to the front of the shoe. Make sure you pick a pair of shoes that match the activity you plan on doing in them and ensure that they have appropriate arch support.

Test your new shoes:

> ➤ Walk on a hard surface
> ➤ Look for wobble on shoe drop
> ➤ View the shoe from the back
> ➤ Bend the shoe the way your foot will bend

While walking you need shoes to handle the heel to toe motion. Your shoes need to protect your feet. Do not forget the inserts!

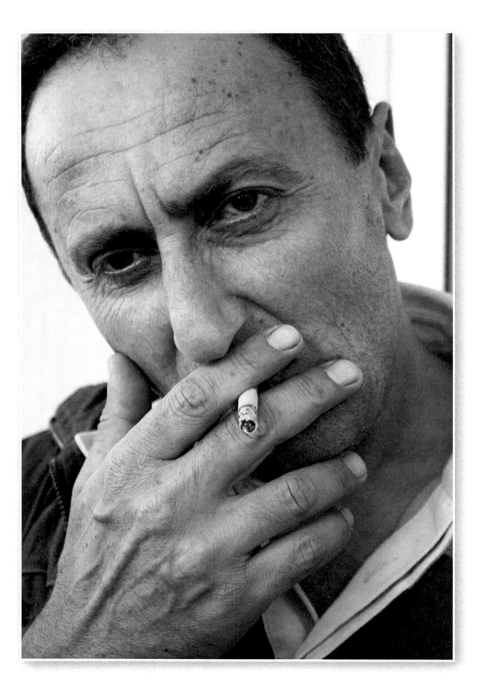

CHAPTER 9

Nicotine and Your Health

Remember that first puff of a cigarette? The wave of nausea, the dizziness, the cough, the lightheadedness? This is the smoker's high. Why do some put the cigarettes down and never pick them up again while others become physically and psychologically addicted?

In spite of it being a known fact that cigarettes cause cancer, heart disease, emphysema, and other diseases, 20 percent of the American population continues to smoke. Globally 4 million people die each year from diseases directly related to tobacco.

In cultures that enjoy a longer life expectancy, the disease, as a result of the accumulation of bodily insult and injury, becomes more apparent. Smokers are 2.7 times more likely to have back pain. Smokers develop low back pain as they get older, with women being more prone than men. Smoking is also blamed for the decay of spinal discs, osteoporosis and failure of spinal fusion surgery.

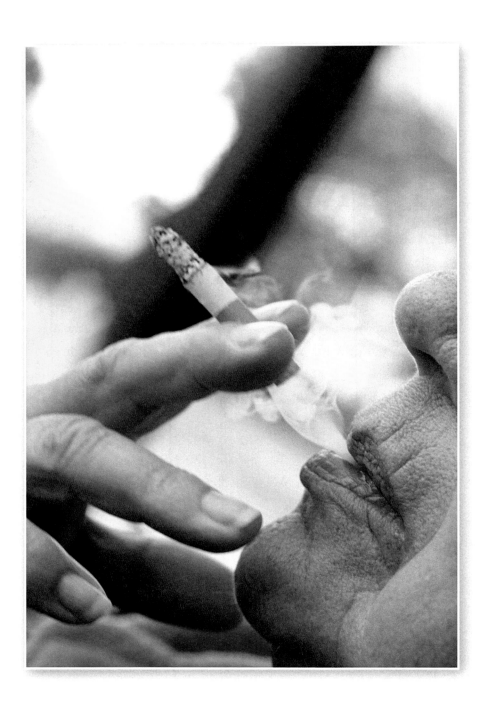

Smoking is responsible for decreased nutrition to the spine due to the carbon monoxide in cigarette smoke. The carbon monoxide sticks to hemoglobin, which is the oxygen carrying part of the blood, and subsequently decreases oxygen supply to all body tissues. Regardless of whether you smoke it, chew it, sniff it or absorb it in a patch, the active substance in tobacco is nicotine. Nicotine, which is the prime chemical in tobacco, increases blood pressure by constricting blood vessels. Nicotine also causes collagen to stop being formed in the center of discs, tendons, ligaments and cartilage. Thus the majority of nonsmokers are able to heal disc lesions and other relatively avascular structures such as tendons, ligaments and cartilage, whereas smokers are unable to heal disc tears and other relatively avascular structures, and have higher rate of unsuccessful fusions.

Cutting down on smoking decreases the chance of developing back pain and the failure of injury healing. After 48 hours of nonsmoking, the nerve endings of your back will start to grow back as a result of the increased blood flow. The cornea of the eye and the intervertebral disc are the only two structures in adult life that do not have a direct blood supply. When smoking cessation occurs, dilatation of the blood vessels and increased blood flow allows for diffusion of nutrients, and results in an increase in oxygen from the bones to the spine to the discs. A disc that is unable to get its nutrition will develop cracks or tears, which will lead to ruptures or herniations.

Your best bet to enjoy good health is to stay active, exercise, and to not smoke or use any other nicotine product.

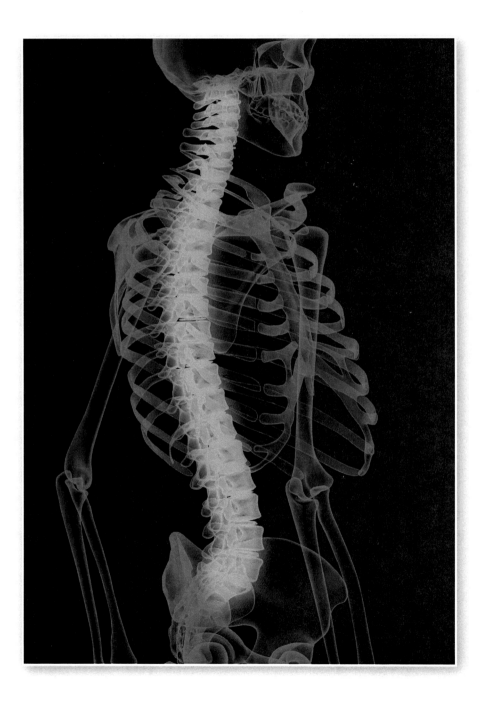

CHAPTER 10

Manipulation

Spinal manipulation is a therapeutic intervention performed on the spinal joints. Hippocrates, the father of medicine, used manipulative techniques. Now chiropractors, osteopathic physicians, occupational therapists and physical therapists most commonly provide spinal manipulation. Orthopedic surgeons are also known to use these techniques when performing closed reductions of fractures and dislocations.

The three phases of spinal manipulation are:

1. Preload or pre-thrust
2. Thrust
3. Resolution

The effects of spinal manipulation are:

➤ Shortened time to recovery
➤ Temporary relief of musculoskeletal pain

- ➤ Temporary increased range of motion
- ➤ Physiologic effects
- ➤ Altered sensorimotor integration

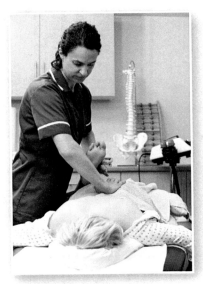

Spinal manipulation may result in symptomatic relief of musculoskeletal pain but may also result in pain or local discomfort, headaches, tiredness, an audible popping sound as gas is released from a joint, or radiating pain. There is a long-held myth that cracking your knuckles damages your joints. People are equally concerned when they hear pops coming from their backs. The facts are that when you pop a joint you stretch the space between the bones. Expanding the joint space creates a negative pressure like a vacuum. The vacuum subsequently sucks in synovial fluid or joint fluid and that forms a bubble. When the bubble collapses you hear a pop.

The spine has two facet joints per spinal level. One can create a number of pops considering that there are seven cervical levels, 12 thoracic levels and five lumbar levels available for popping. Popping can be created by bending, twisting, or chiropractic mobilization. Some people find popping to be very pleasurable while others find it to be painful. Current opinion is that a little is okay, but excessive mobilization of joints on a frequent basis may accelerate degenerative arthritis. Catastrophic events such as cervical artery dissections have been reported, thus manipulation of the neck in the elderly should be carefully weighed.

CHAPTER 11

Mental game

In order to recover from an injury there are three action steps you should take.

The three key elements for healing yourself after an injury are:

1. Use good pain science data
2. Remember that sometimes less is more
3. Have a carefully constructed rehabilitation program

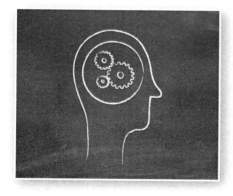

Paying attention to these three elements helps prevent re-injury and allows for a steady, progressive recovery. When you sustain an injury your brain tells the injured part of the body that there is pain, to stop and protect that area of the body to allow it to recover. Once the injury has healed the brain has a tendency to hold on to that signal and keep your body in a similar environment to the one you were injured in. Thus the brain feels your body still hurts in spite of it not actually hurting anymore. This is often described as phantom pain. In order to correct the situation you must perform controlled, thoughtful movements so as to break the circuit of phantom pain. In order to prevent re-injury you must perform slow, steady and increasing amounts of exercise. Overdoing it will result in a setback. For the athlete trying to get better faster, a less is more approach is often prudent. Carefully constructing a plan for recovery will avoid setbacks. By consulting your physician or physical therapist or exercise physiologist/trainer you may progress safely through the recovery program.

How to apply the principle:

1. Plan on doing a bit of everything that you had planned for the day
2. Test your movements before excessively loading them
3. Preparation, body and brain warm-up are important

A study by Harte and colleagues evaluated how beta-endorphin, corticotropin-releasing hormone and cortisol from the hypothalamic-pituitary-adrenocortical area affect mood changes. The authors took elite runners and highly trained meditators. They studied the metabolic differences between the runners and meditators, and evaluated mood change as a result of both activities. With running there was an elevation of beta-endorphins and corticotropin-releasing hormone. With meditation there was an elevation of corticotropin-releasing hormone. It should be noted that there was no difference between the two groups. This study demonstrated that running can aid in pain control and mood improvement, whereas meditation is able to result in only mood enhancement.

Some people have a history of depression, anxiety, stress, fear and mis-understanding of pain. These conditions stimulate the spinal cord to start a central amplification process. Depression and anxiety can be treated successfully with medications and cognitive behavioral therapy. Exercise is an effective treatment for depression. Meditation, yoga, stress management exercises are all helpful for managing stress.

Various areas of the brain are responsible for interacting to create these symptoms. The best pain rehabilitation program understands and ad-dresses these situations. It becomes extremely important for an accurate diagnosis prior to the formulation of a treatment plan.

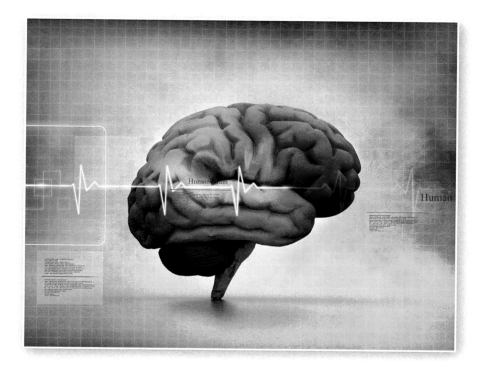

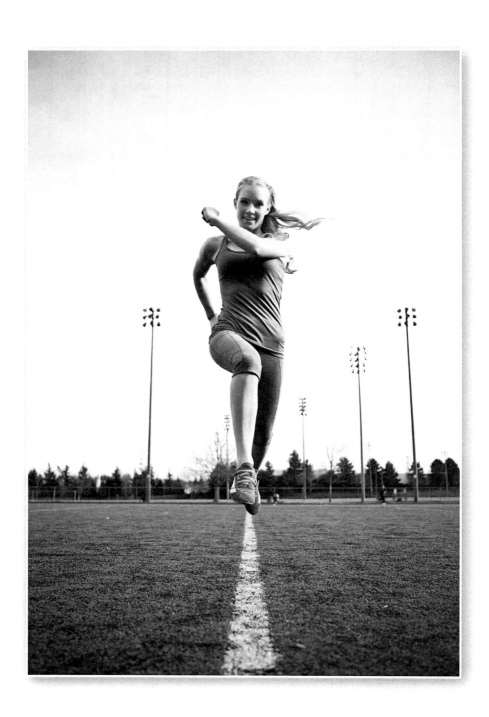

CHAPTER 12

The Future

In order to reap the benefits of a hard workout, your body needs to learn to recover. The inescapable part of the training cycle — **stress, recovery, adaptation** — is what separates the recreational athlete from the professional athlete. Professional athletes seem to be devoted to ice baths, compression garments and other aids. The inflammation and soreness that you feel the morning after a workout is telling you that your body needs to adapt. Recently, coaches and trainers have suggested that athletes need to adopt different strategies at different points in their training cycle for recovery. If you are in a period of heavy training where the goal is to increase fitness, then you should minimize the use of ice baths, other aids and antioxidants. Yet as you approach an important competition, you should use recovery aids such as ice baths, antioxidants and others to recover your full strength prior to competition. This same mantra may be applied to any injury, illness or disease — **insult, recovery, adaptation**. In the future there will be many more discoveries that will allow improvement of injuries, illnesses or diseases. As such there will be a continual evolution of discovery, learning, application and evolution. The subtle shift of how we think is important in an accelerated recovery program.

With the introduction of new technologies, new medicines, re-engineering of old technology with new applications, and better understanding of the biology of injury we are seeing a more rapid return to activities. Now all we have to do is unlock the immortality of the cell.

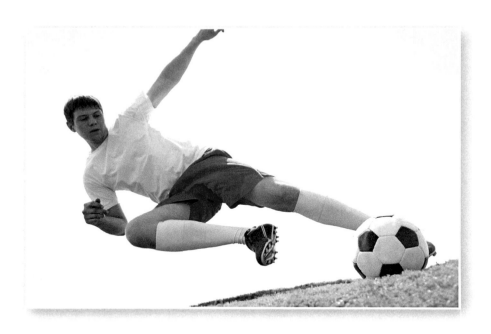

Glossary

Ablation – The removal of an organ, abnormal growth or harmful area from the body by a mechanical means

Accelerated Postoperative Recovery (APR) – Program of treatment used after surgery to accelerate recovery and decrease complications

Accelerated recovery program – Technique used to enhance the body's ability to recover itself after injury, illness or surgery

Acquired immune deficiency syndrome (AIDS) – A condition caused by an infection from the human immunodeficiency virus (HIV)

Activities of daily living (ADLs) – Refers to people's daily self-care activities

Addison's disease – A chronic condition brought on by the failure of the adrenal glands

Anabolic steroids – Synthetic derivatives of the male hormone testosterone

Apoptosis – A natural process of self-destruction of a cell, which is also known as programmed cell death

Atherosclerosis – The buildup of fats, cholesterol and other substances in and on your artery walls, or plaque, that results in the restriction of blood flow

Autonomic dysreflexia (hyperreflexia) – A reaction of the autonomic or involuntary nervous system to overstimulation that is a potentially life-threatening condition

Autonomic nervous system – Division of peripheral nervous system that controls the function of internal organs

Beta-endorphin – A potent hormone that is released by the body's anterior pituitary gland in response to pain, trauma, exercise or other forms of stress and is known as the body's own pain killer

Blastocyte – An undifferentiated embryonic cell. Cells that are derived from the inner cell mass of the blastocyst are known as embryonic stem cells

Body mass index (BMI) – A formula used to calculate a person's body fat content based on his or her weight and height

Calorie – A unit of food energy that is approximately the amount of energy needed to raise the temperature of 1 kg of water by 1 C

Caudal – The anatomic route meaning inferior or below another structure in order to gain access to an anatomic area

Cell senescence – The gradual deterioration or aging of a cell

Cerebrovascular accident (CVA) – The sudden death of brain cells due to a lack of oxygen when the blood flow to the brain is impaired by either blockage or rupture of an artery in the brain. More commonly known as a stroke.

Complete injury – Where there is a total lack of sensory and motor function below the level of injury

Contamination – The unwanted pollution of something by another substance

Corticotropin-releasing hormone – A peptide hormone involved in the stress response

Cortisol – A steroid hormone produced by the adrenal cortex and released by the body in response to stress and low blood glucose

Creatine – A nitrogenous organic acid that helps to supply energy to all cells in the body, especially muscle, as it increases the formation of adenosine triphosphate (ATP)

CT scan – Computed tomography scan

Deep vein thrombosis (DVT) – A condition where a blood clot forms in a vein deep inside a part of the body

Disability – A consequence of an impairment that may be physical, cognitive, mental, sensory, emotional, developmental or some combination of these

Discectomy – The surgical removal of a herniated disc that is putting pressure on a spinal nerve or the spinal cord

Doctor – The holder of an accredited doctoral graduate degree

Dual X-ray absorbtiometry (DXA) – The preferred technique for measuring bone mineral density or soft bone

Durotomy – The incision of the dura mater or the tissue surrounding the spinal cord or nerve root

EMG – Electromyography study

Epidural Steroid Injection (ESI) – A medical route of administration where a drug or medicine is placed above the dura where the membrane surrounding the spinal cord or nerve

Epithelialization – A component of wound healing where there is a growth of epithelial or skin cells over an injured area

Fibroblastic repair – A phase in wound healing where fibroblast cells begin activity leading to scar formation

Foraminotomy – The enlargement of the spinal nerve hole or foramina in order to relieve pressure on a spinal nerve

Fragility fracture – Any fall from a standing height or less that results in a fracture

Handicap – A disadvantage that makes achievement unusually difficult. It results when a disability or impairment limits or prevents the fulfillment of a role

Heat exhaustion – A heat-related illness that occurs after exposure to high temperature

Heatstroke – A condition caused by your body overheating due to prolonged exposure to a high temperature and represents a medical emergency

Hibiclens (Mölnlycke Health Care, Gothenburg, Sweden) – A 4 percent chlorhexidine gluconate solution (CHG) that acts as an antiseptic and antimicrobial skin cleanser used to prevent infection

Human growth hormone (HGH) – Produced in the pituitary gland and helps to regulate body composition, body fluids, muscle and bone growth, sugar and fat metabolism, and possibly heart function; used by some as a performance-enhancing drug to build muscle, improve athletic performance and decrease aging

Hypermetabolism – The body's state of an increased rate of metabolic activity

Hypometabolism – The body's state of decreased rate of metabolic activity

Impact (Nestlé Health Sciences) – A nutritional supplement with arginine, omega-3 fatty acids and nucleotides to help meet the immune response in a postoperative or post injury requirement need

Impairment – A medical evaluation that determines the state of being diminished, weakened or damaged either physically or mentally

Incomplete injury – Where the ability of the spinal cord to convey messages to and from the brain is not completely lost

Inflammation – The process where the white blood cells and tissue fluids are delivered to an injured tissue

Insulin-like growth factor-1 (IGF-1) – A protein hormone necessary for proper growth in children and used by athletes to accelerate recover, but significantly increases the risk of cancer development

Interspinous device – A new spinal implant that is placed between the vertebral bodies spinous processes for the treatment of lumbar spinal degenerative disease

Laminectomy – The surgical removal of the bony posterior arch of a spinal vertebra in order to access the spinal canal

Laminotomy – The partial removal of the bony posterior arch of the spinal vertebra in order to access the spinal canal

Level of injury – The determination by a physician of the location of the spinal cord injury

LLLT – Low-level laser therapy

MEP – Motor evoked potentials

Metabolic equivalent of tasks (METs) – The metabolic unit used to quantify the intensity of physical activity; defined as the ratio of the metabolic rate during exercise to the metabolic rate at rest

Microdiscectomy – Or microdecompression spine surgery, is where through a small incision a small amount of bone may be removed from the spine in order to gain access and relieve pressure on a nerve

Microgram – A microgram (mcg) is one thousandth of a milligram.

Morbid obesity – When excess body fat becomes a danger to your overall health

MRI – Magnetic resonance imaging

NCV- Nerve conduction velocity study

Neurogenic shock – The physiological response to shock that results in low blood pressure, occasionally a slowed heart rate and is attributed to the disruption of the autonomic pathways within the spinal cord

Nonsteroidal anti-inflammatory drug (NSAIDS) – A class of drugs that provides pain-killing, fever-reducing, and anti-inflammatory effects

Obesity – A condition where you have too much body fat for your height or have an elevated body mass index (BMI)

Osteoarthritis – The "wear and tear" arthritis; occurs when the protective cartilage on the ends of the bones wears down over time

Osteopenia – A mild thinning of bone mass that weakens bone structure

Osteoporosis – A marked thinning of bone mass that weakens bone structure

Paraplegia – An impairment in the motor or sensory function to the lower extremities

Phantom pain – A perception experienced relating to a limb or organ that is not physically part of your body

Photobiomodulation – Also known as low-level laser therapy, is the exposure of a low-level laser light or light emitting diode that stimulates cellular function leading to a beneficial clinical effect

Pilates – A physical fitness system developed by Joseph Pilates that is intended to strengthen the body and mind

Platelet-rich plasma (PRP) – Blood plasma that has been enriched with platelets and is used to concentrate growth factors that are important in the healing of injuries

Pronation – A rotation of the hand or foot to a position of either palm or sole down, respectively

Pulmonary embolism (PE) – A blood clot that has migrated to the lungs; results in restricted blood flow inside the lungs, and results in poor oxygen exchange

Quadriplegia – An impairment in the motor or sensory function to the upper and lower extremities

Radiculopathy – A pinched nerve in the spine

RICE principle – The immediate treatment of any soft tissue injury or skeletal muscle injury through rest, ice, compression and elevation

SOMI – Suboccipital mandibular orthosis

Spinal cord injury – Any damage to the spinal cord or nerves that causes changes in sensation, strength or other body functions

Spinal fusion – A surgery to permanently connect two or more spinal vertebra so there is no movement

Spinal shock – A term that relates to the loss of all neurological activity, including loss of motor, sensory, reflex and autonomic function below the level of injury

Spondylolisthesis – A condition of the spine where one bone slides forward over another bone below it

SSEP – Somatosensory evoked potentials

Stem cell – An undifferentiated, or blank, cell that has the potential to develop into other cells serving many different functions in many parts of the body

Supination – A rotation of the hand or foot to a position of either palm or sole up, respectively

TENS – Transcutaneous electrical nerve stimulation

Transforaminal – Route going through a foramen of the spine

Transitional mobility assister – Any device that allows a more efficient use of energy for locomotion (cane, crutches, wheelchair, scooter, etc.)

Translaminar – Route going across or through a lamina of the spine

U.S. Food and Drug administration (FDA) – A federal agency of the United States Department of Health and Human Services that is responsible for protecting the public health by regulating food, dietary supplements, tobacco, prescription and over-the-counter pharmaceutical medications, vaccines, blood transfusions, bio-pharmaceuticals, medical devices, animal foods and feed, veterinary products, and electromagnetic radiation emitting devices

Vertebrectomy – The removal of a spinal vertebra

Vitamin – An organic compound or vital nutrient that the body requires in a limited amount

Yoga – A physical, mental and spiritual practice that originated in India

References

Anderson, M., S. Hall and M. Martin. *Sports Injury Management.* 2nd ed. Philadelphia: Lippincott Williams and Wilkins, 2000. Print.

"Ankle Sprains: How to Speed Your Recovery." *Down East Orthopedics.* American Orthopaedic Society for Sports Medicine, 2008. Web. **www.downeastorthopedics.com/assets/Ankle-Sprains.pdf**.

Archer, Todd, "Aikman offers cautionary tale for Romo." ESPN, 23 Dec. 2013. Web. **http://espn.go.com/blog/dallas-cowboys/post/_/id/4722370/troy-aikman-offers-cautionary-tale -for-romo**.

Arden, C.L., N. F. Taylor, J.A. Feller and K.E. Webster. "A systematic review of psychological factors associated with returning to sports following injury." *British Journal of Sports Medicine* 47 (2013): 1120-1126.

Bahr, Roald and Sverre Maehlum. *Clinical Guide to Sports Injuries.* Champaign: Human Kinetics, 2004. Print.

Bell, Jarrett, "When it comes to back trouble, Aikman can relate to Romo." *USA Today Sports*. USA Today, 10 Dec. 2014. Web. **www.usatoday.com/story/sports/nfl/cowboys/2014/12/09/bell-aikman-can-relate-to-romo-and-his-back-trouble/20167621**.

Brady, James, "Tony Romo suffered collarbone fracture, will miss rest of season." SBNation, 27 Nov. 2015. Web. **www.sbnation.com/nfl/2015/11/26/9805398/tony-romo-injury-cowboys-panthers-matt-cassel**.

Brouwer, P.A., et al. "Percutaneous laser disk decompression versus conventional microdiscectomy in sciatica: a randomized controlled trial." *The Spine Journal* 15.5 (2015): 857-865.

Brown, Suzanne, "Klaus Obermeyer still skiing, yodeling, and making snow wear." *The Denver Post*, 2 Feb. 2013. Web. **www.denverpost.com/ci_22503203/klaus-obermeyer-still-skiing-yodeling-and-making-snow**.

Campbell, Barbara J. "Calcium, Nutrition, and Bone Health." *Orthoinfo*. AAOS, July 2012. Web. **http://orthoinfo.aaos.org/topic.cfm?topic=A00317**.

Cotler, H.B. "A NASA discovery has current applications in orthopedics." *Current Orthopaedic Practice* 26.1 (2015): 72-74.

Cotler, H.B., R.T. Chow, M.R. Hamblin and J. Carroll. "The use of low level laser therapy (LLLT) for musculoskeletal pain." *MOJ Orthopedics & Rheumatology* 2.5 (2015): 1-8.

Crane, Kristine. "Enhanced recovery: improving patient surgical experience." U.S. News and World Report, 4 Feb. 2015. Web. **http://health.usnews.com/ health-news/patient-advice/articles/2015/02/04/ enhanced-recovery-improving-patients-surgical-experience**.

Fitzgerald, Matt, "Tiger Woods Injury: Updates on Golfer's Recovery from Back Surgery," Bleacher Report, 2015. Web. **http://bleacherreport.com/articles/2581138-tiger-woods-injury-updates-on-golfers-recovery-from-back-surgery**.

Ford, Bonnie, "Landis admits doping, accuses Lance," ESPN, 21 May 2010. Web. **http://espn.go.com/figure-skating/cycling/news/ story?id=5203604**.

Garbutt, G., M.G. Boocock, T. Reilly and J.D. Troup. "Running speed and spinal shrinkage in runners with and without back pain." *Medicine & Science in Sports & Exercise* 22.6 (1990): 769-772.

Gay, Jason, "This is 40. Tiger Woods Gets Closer to the Rest of Us." The Wall Street Journal, 2 Dec. 2015. Web. **www.wsj.com/ articles/this-is-40-tiger-woods-gets-closer-to-the-rest-of-us-1449098824**.

Hagen, K.B., G. Jamtvedt, G. Hilde and M.F. Winnem. "The updated Cochrane review of bed rest for low back pain and sciatica." *Spine (Phila Pa 1976)* 30.5 (2005): 542-546. PubMed 9971865.

Harte, J.L., G.H. Eifert and R. Smith. "The effect of running and meditation on beta-endorphin, corticotropin-releasing hormone and cortisol in plasma, and on mood." *Biological Psychology* 40.3 (1995): 251-265.

Hubbard, T.J. and C.R. Denegar. "Does cryotherapy improve outcomes with soft tissue injury?" *Journal of Athletic Training* 39.3 (2004): 278-279.

Hupin, D., et al. "Even low dose to moderate to vigorous physical activity reduces mortality by 22% in adults aged equal to or greater than 60 years: a systematic review and meta-analysis." *British Journal of Sports Medicine* doi:10.1136/bjsports-2014-094306.

Hutchinson, A. "Fitness: Ice baths, antioxidant supplements not always the best route to recovery." The Globe and Mail, 23 Aug. 2015. Web. **www.theglobeandmail.com/life/health-and-fitness/fitness/ice-baths-antioxidant-supplements-not-always-the-best-route-to-recovery/article26052576**.

Kelly, Frank B. "Platelet-Rich Plasma (PRP)." *OrthoInfo*. AAOS, Sept. 2011. Web. **http://orthoinfo.aaos.org/topic.cfm?topic=A00648**.

Lambert, Ellen, "Does Wearing a Waist-Trimmer Belt Help You Burn Belly Fat While Your Exercise?" Houston Chronicle, 2015. Web. **http://livehealthy.chron.com/wearing-waisttrimmer-belt-burn-belly-fat-exercise-9314.html**.

Manini, T.M., et al. "Daily activity energy expenditure and mortality among older adults." *Journal of the American Medical Association* 296.2 (2006): 171-179.

Murphy, Jen, "At 95, a Lifelong Skier Says the Source of His Vitality is His Workout." The Wall Street Journal, 30 Nov. 2015. Web. **www.wsj.com/articles/at-95-a-lifelong-skiier-says-the-source-of-his-vitality-is-his-workout-1448899633.**

Neumann, Janice. "For seniors, any exercise may be better than none." Reuters, 21 Aug. 2015. Web. **www.reuters.com/article/us-health-elderly-fitness-mortality-idUSKCN0QQ1M620150821.**

Oldmeadow, L.B., E.R. Edwards, L.A. Kimmel, et al. "No rest for the wounded: early ambulation after hip surgery accelerates recovery." *ANZ Journal of Surgery* 76.7 (2006): 607-611. PubMed #16813627.

Patrick, C.A., et al. "Lack of effectiveness of bed rest for sciatica." *The New England Journal of Medicine* 340.6 (1999): 418-423. PubMed#9971865.

Severson, Dana, "How Does the Trimmer Belt Help You to Lose Belly Weight?" Livestrong.com, 16 April 2015. Web. **www.livestrong.com/article/404277-how-does-the-trimmer-belt-help-you-to-lose-belly-weight.**

Sobel, Jason and Bob Harig, "Tiger Woods undergoes back surgery to remove disk fragment," ESPN, 19 Sept. 2015. Web. **http://espn.go.com/golf/story/_/id/13687070/tiger-woods-undergoes-another-back-surgery.**

Sorrenti, S.J. "Achilles tendon rupture: effective early mobilization in rehabilitation after surgical repair." *Foot & Ankle International* 27.6 (2006): 407-410. PubMed#16764705.

Storrs, Carina. "Is Platelet-Rich Plasma and Effective Healing Therapy?" Scientific American, 18 Dec. 2009. Web. **www.scientificamerican.com/article/platelet-rich-plasma-therapy-dennis-cardone-sports-medicine-injury**.

Vigelsoe, Andreas, et al. "Six weeks' aerobic training after two weeks' immobilization restores leg lean mass and aerobic capacity but does not fully rehabilitate leg strength in young and older men." *Journal of Rehabilitation Medicine* (2015) doi: 10.2340/16501977-1961.

Wilson, Jacque, "Lance Armstrong's doping drugs." CNN, 18 Jan. 2013. Web. **www.cnn.com/2013/01/15/health/armstrong-ped-explainer**.

Wilson, Stephen, "Johnson, Jones, Armstrong: Sport's doping hall of shame." *The Big Story*. AP News, 10 Nov. 2015. Web. **http://bigstory.ap.org/article/0151ea607e8143a8bc50d504a0b858fe/johnson-jones-armstrong-sports-doping-hall-shame**.

Zelman, Kathleen, "The Olympic Diet of Michael Phelps." WebMD, 13 Aug. 2008. **www.webmd.com/diet/20080813/the-olympic-diet-of-michael-phelps**.

Index

G

Gyrotonic, 124

H

Heart disease, 22, 28, 85, 89, 110, 135

Hot tub, 68

Human growth hormone (HGH), 56, 151

Hypertension, 28, 53, 57, 58, 63, 89

I

Insulin-like growth factor-1 (IGF-1), 56, 152

L

Laser surgery, 96

Low-level laser therapy (LLLT), 33, 72

M

Massage, 33, 69, 70, 103

Minimally invasive surgery, 92

Muscle relaxers, 49

N

Narcotics, 27, 40, 48, 49, 51

Nonsteroidal anti-inflammatory drugs (NSAIDs), 53

O

Obesity, 87, 89, 90, 153

Oral steroids, 53, 54

Osteoarthritis, 71, 73, 83, 86, 89, 122, 153

Osteoporosis, 21, 22, 54, 135, 153

P

Phantom pain, 142, 154

Pulmonary emboli (PE), 29

R

RICE, 31-33, 42, 103, 154

S

T

W

Y

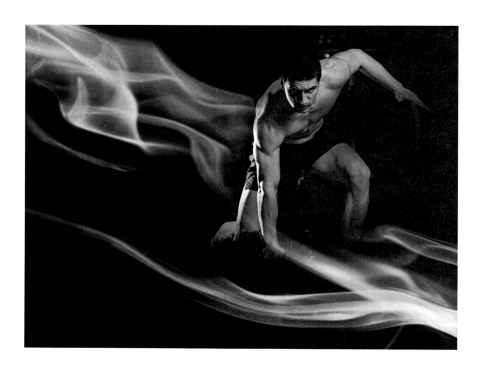